PRAISE FOR
HER RIGHT TO KNOW

"This is a true story of a courageous woman rendered blind because a drug company hid the truth, and a courageous young lawyer who through our justice system heroically battled overwhelming odds to prove it. It puts the reader, whether lawyer or layperson, in the courtroom at the counsel table as well as in the jury box. It is a significant and inspiring book which all who use the American health system, especially women, should read. They owe a debt of gratitude to Sal Liccardo."

—William Whitehurst, Past President of The International Academy of Trial Lawyers, The Texas Trial Lawyers Association, & Registered Pharmacist

"A courageous true story written by a highly regarded, esteemed trial lawyer. This book reveals a courageous trial lawyer and an equally courageous young woman, as his client, search for the truth about the "Pill." It further demonstrates the power of a jury to make the world a safer place. Having spent my life supporting the right to trial by jury, I heartily encourage reading this enlightening book."

—Ron Rouda, J.D., Past National President of the American Board of Trial Advocates (ABOTA)

"An enjoyable, compelling, well rendered read! It reads like a novel . . . enough plot twists to make it riveting."

—John Lenahan, M.D.

"A moving real time story that reads like a novel."

—Thaddeus Whalen, Ph.D., Professor Emeritus
in Economics, Santa Clara University

HER RIGHT TO KNOW

HER RIGHT TO KNOW

Published by TLLF Publishing

Book Design by Lisa Abellera

ISBN 978-0-5785802-9-6 (paperback)

ISBN 978-0-5785803-0-2 (ebook)

Library of Congress Control Number: 2019914644

First Edition: October 2019

HER RIGHT TO KNOW

One Trial Lawyer's Search for the Truth About the "Pill"

SAL LICCARDO

To Michelle and Dennis for their enormous courage in seeing this case through to its end, and to my wife, Laura, for her moral support and willingness to share the risk.

Author's Note

This is a true story.

The substance has not been changed. Although the entire trial was transcribed, the record of it unfortunately has been lost or destroyed by the time of this writing. Fortunately for me, the Appellate Court opinion, and my extensive opening and closing briefs, along with miscellaneous pleadings and published newspaper articles were preserved and available for my reference. Much of the dialog was reconstructed from the substance stated in the foregoing documents and some are reproduced from memory. In some places I abbreviated and/or modified the dialog to make it more readable. The majority of the real-life characters are unfortunately deceased, but I was assisted by the reliable memories of particularly my clients, Dennis and Michelle, as well as my wife, Laura. To protect the privacy of the jurors, aliases are used. To protect other's privacy, their full name was not used.

I am the sole writer and author of this book.

I consider trial by Jury as the only anchor ever yet imagined by man, by which a government can be held to the principles of its constitution.

—Thomas Jefferson

Contents

Author's Note   i

Introduction   1

Chapter 1   3
   A Mysterious Nightmare Comes To Life

Chapter 2   21
   A Search For The Mysterious Cause

Chapter 3   30
   The Story Unfolds

Chapter 4   44
   Digging for Gold

Chapter 5   60
   A Black Cloud on the Horizon

Chapter 6   77
   The Jury

Chapter 7   88
   Trial Begins
       Donald G. Harris, M.D.   95
       Herbert Ley, M.D.   100
       Robert McCleery, M.D.   101

Chapter 8   108

The Truth Unfolds

Jerome Bettman, M.D.   108

John Altshuler, M.D.   115

John Leissring, M.D.   121

Martin Overton, M.D.   124

J. Ray Van Meter, M.D.   129

Larry Gossack, M.D.   132

Thomas Preston   137

Alice   138

Dennis Ahearn   140

Michelle Ahearn   143

CHAPTER 9   150

Johnson & Johnson Fights Back

Martin Kosmin, M.D.   151

Phillip Lippe, M.D.   161

Richard Sogg, M.D.   168

CHAPTER 10   180

Big Pharma Fires Its Big Guns

Bruce Ostler, M.D.   180

William McCabe, M.D.   185

Miss Yue   192

Ernest Page, M.D.   193

Joseph Goldzeirher, M.D.   198

Arnold Cronk, M.D.   204

CHAPTER 11   216

Summing Up the Truth

CHAPTER 12   244
    The Verdict

CHAPTER 13   260
    The 13th Juror

CHAPTER 14   276
    Three Justices Weigh In

CHAPTER 15   289
    The California Supreme Court—The Final Answer

Epilogue   296

Afterword   308

Newspaper Articles   312

Appendix A   338

Acknowledgments   341

About The Author   343

INTRODUCTION

In the '60's and '70's millions of young women—wives, mothers, sisters, daughters, suffered heart attacks, strokes, blindness, paralysis, and even death from a cause unknown to them! Why? This is the true story of a young woman who suffered sudden catastrophic blindness. It is the story how this tenacious woman, together with twelve courageous jurors, used the rule of law in a search for the truth.

Every human being has the right to know of any potential serious harm to their body from any product they consume, whether prescription drugs, medical devices, or food for the table. No industry has the right to take that decision away from us, particularly Big Pharma. The duty to warn of known risks is imbedded in the American Law of Torts.

Amazingly, many Americans are not familiar with the term "tort" which comes from the French word meaning a "wrongful injury." The essence of American Tort Law is to make wrongdoers accountable and responsible for the wrongful injuries they cause, regardless of their power or size. This duty to warn of known risks should be implemented at every level of our industrial society. But it has not been so in the past nor is it so in the present.

This is another chapter in the war against corporate greed. Fought from courthouse to courthouse—trial by trial—throughout this great nation, its purpose is not only the pursuit of justice alone, but equally to save American lives and reduce human suffering. This story depicts only one of millions of such battles fought in this war.

CHAPTER 1
A MYSTERIOUS NIGHTMARE COMES TO LIFE

It was early November, a typical beautiful fall day in San Jose, California. As I momentarily looked up from reviewing boring depositions in a pending case, I noticed through my office window the beauty of the fall leaves from the trees lining The Alameda. I was anxious to finish and leave for home to enjoy a run with my kids before dark when my younger brother, Len, poked his nose into my office, asking if I had a moment to discuss something. Such casual interruptions were common and welcomed in our small, boutique law firm in 1969.

"Sure, Len, what's up?" I replied. Len handled our business and criminal defense practice.

"I just saw Dennis Ahearn," he said. "He needed some legal assistance in starting his own practice as a structural engineer. He recently left the engineering firm where he'd worked for several years. Dennis says this has been his dream for a long time, and he didn't want to wait years until his old firm decided to place his name on the door."

Dennis and his wife, Michelle were friends from my school years of growing up in San Jose. Dennis and I attended the same high school in our valley, Bellarmine College Prep. Although he was a couple years behind me in class, we still knew one another. In the early years of his career, Dennis taught engineering at my alma mater, Santa Clara University. My brother Len and Dennis were quite close friends. Michelle was a close friend to my godmother's daughter, so we would see each other on occasion, but it had been some time.

Len continued, "I have some very sad news. Dennis told me Michelle has suddenly become blind due to a strep throat. I told him he should discuss the circumstances with you since that sounded awfully strange to me."

I found it unbelievable with the medical experience and education I had accumulated, that anyone could become permanently blind from *just* a strep throat.

"Len, I can't believe a strep throat would cause blindness. There had to be something else going on. The next time you see Dennis, ask if he and Michelle would be willing to talk to me about what happened. People just don't go blind from strep throats."

"I'll be seeing them next week. We have our investment club meeting and I'll tell him then you'd like to talk to them about Michelle's sudden blindness."

I grabbed my coat, left the office and began my drive home. I couldn't get it out of my mind—how strange that someone would go blind from a strep throat. I couldn't believe a doctor could make such a strange connection; I was very puzzled.

Though my formal education did not include any significant medical courses, having received a bachelor's degree in political science and a law degree at Santa Clara University. I, did, however, marry a nurse.

Driving home, I reflected on our early years of law practice when my partner, Richard (Dick) Caputo and I, pursued our joint interest in learning as much medicine as possible. Three nights a week after a full day of work, we drove 50 miles to the University of California Medical School in San Francisco, to pursue an evening medical school program involving courses in anatomy, physiology (the physical functioning of the human body), pharmacology (the effect of prescription drugs on the human body) and more. We were convinced that any lawyer who specialized in personal injury work, as we were doing, must be well grounded in medicine to be able to evaluate the merits of a case, particularly to competently examine and cross-examine physicians within various specialties of medicine.

A further coincidental advantage in our accumulation of medical knowledge occurred when Dick and I asked two close friends and clients, who happened to be pathologists, Paul Vincent, M.D. and William (Bill) Siegel, M.D., to join us on occasional mid-week ski trips to the California Sierras. For over three hours each way, as we drove Dick and I would take advantage of their medical expertise in brainstorming current cases. They had an interest in the legal issues raised in our cases as well. Their ability to determine medical causation in cases was invaluable.

On one of these trips, Paul suggested, "Why don't you guys scrub in on an autopsy with me or Bill? It'll be a great learning experience for you guys."

I jumped at the opportunity.

"Let me know when your next autopsy is scheduled, and I'll try to be there." I subsequently scrubbed in on several autopsies with each of them. When you see, touch and feel an anatomical structure in a cadaver, you never forget it. This method certainly beat trying to understand two-dimension medical illustrations in medical textbooks.

Dick and I also regularly attended weekend medical programs designed to educate personal injury lawyers. The focus of these programs was primarily on orthopedic and neurological injuries that commonly arose in auto collisions, falls, workplace injuries and more.

✍

As Len told me of Michelle's blindness from a mere strep throat, immediately came to mind an unusual medical lecture Dick and I had attended a few months earlier. It focused on vascular disorders, particularly blood clotting risks such as blindness. What we heard, we did not expect. This lecture was given by a dedicated physician, Dr. J. Harold Williams, M.D., LL.B., who had practiced medicine several years in California before becoming a lawyer.

Dr. Williams gave an unusually dramatic, eloquent lecture that day, a surprisingly emotional talk for a physician, passionate about a subject to which he had devoted several years of his professional life. Harold was seeking an answer to a spooky question.

He raised the question, "Why are so many women of childbearing age ending up in hospitals and morgues from diagnosed blood clotting disorders today at levels not seen before? As I reviewed hospital records on each woman, I looked for medical evidence common to the vast majority of these young female patients. I surprisingly discovered that at the time of their illness or lethal event in which each had suffered a blood clotting disorder, most of these young women had coincidentally been on *oral contraceptives, the "Pill."*

The medical evidence he presented to support his conclusion of a causal relationship between the "Pill" and blood clotting was extremely impressive and somewhat persuasive. For those reasons, I found it quite memorable. Most striking was the total absence of such knowledge at that time among practicing physicians prescribing the "Pill," as well as the public at large.

✑

Though Dick and I thought Harold made sense, the rest of the world was not with us. Our country was a very different place in the 1960's. America faced a world of many horrible fears—the assassination of the President of the United States, a war in Vietnam that ultimately cost over 50,000 American lives and over 200,000 wounded, fears of global annihilation from a Russian initiated nuclear war, a civil rights uprising in the South involving outrageous human rights tragedies perpetrated upon black Americans, and last, but certainly not least, the fear the entire world would face *massive starvation from overpopulation!*

This fear of mass starvation from overpopulation was soon to disappear in the mid to late 1960's as science and Big Pharma came to the rescue with the discovery of the previously unknown ingredients that made Oral Contraceptives possible, i.e., the chemical synthetic for estrogen, "ethinyl estradiol." The "Pill" immediately became overwhelmingly popular worldwide and the consumer demand for the "Pill" exploded accordingly. With a stroke of a pen physicians could save the world from potential doom and gloom from overpopulation. A woman could "safely" avoid pregnancy by merely taking a once-a-day pill with the belief there were no significant risks as broadly disseminated by the pharmaceutical manufacturers in their massive advertising. They conceded to only a "few minor side effects." Of course, the pharmaceutical companies selling this product were reaping in a fortune in sales and profits, while their stock price soared on the world security exchanges, and CEOs became richer and richer.

∽

In his lecture, Harold pointed out, "Pharmaceutical manufacturers design, publish and distribute a variety of patient booklets for women's consumption. They promote the 'Pill' as 'safe,' 'well-tolerated,' causing only 'minor discomforts.' They go so far as to represent that there is no medical evidence '*whatsoever*' to substantiate fears of harm from taking the 'Pill.' For more than 15 years of marketing the 'Pill,' not a single morsel of warning has emanated from the pharmaceutical industry that the oral contraceptive might cause blood clots in certain women which could result in stroke, heart attack, paralysis, brain damage, blindness or even death. Unknown to the public, the number of young childbearing age female victims is soaring worldwide."

He noted a handful of early lawsuits had been filed, but the evidence presented in the courtroom had failed to convince juries that the "Pill" had anything to do with blood clots causing injuries or death. Harold indicated he had personally participated, as a trial lawyer, in some of those losing cases.

Listening to Harold's lecture, my trial experience enabled me to recognize the cold fact that the public was not ready to accept such an uncomfortable conclusion—that there might be problems with the "Pill," regardless of the medical and legal evidence to the contrary. After all, the "Pill" gave prescribing physicians the opportunity to become saviors of the world from ultimate starvation and not merely an alternative to avoid pregnancy.

I now asked myself, so how did a perfectly healthy 29-year-old wife and mother become blind for life from a mere strep throat? Could the "Pill" have somehow played a role in her blindness? A search for the truth through Michelle's case began to unfold and unravel this medical mystery.

The next week, Len stepped into my office saying, "Sal, I spoke to Dennis and they'll call you for an appointment to discuss Michelle's blindness."

"Good."

⚬∕⌀

A few days later, Michelle called and made an appointment for Dennis and her to meet with me. I subsequently learned they agreed to meet more out of curiosity as to what I might have to say, than any real interest or desire in pursuing litigation against anyone. They were not litigious people. In fact, both were philosophically averse to becoming involved in any type of litigation. Dennis, a 30-year-old successful structural engineer had just left his employment to start his own professional practice out of his home and did not want to complicate his life with a lawsuit. Michelle, a blind homemaker raising their three small children, ages 2, 5, and 8, also working for Dennis as his secretary, didn't need to complicate her life either. She further acted as his receptionist handling all his phone calls. She was an accomplished typist managing all of the typing work for Dennis' new company despite her blindness.

In my many previous social contacts with each of them, I found them to be very pleasant and enjoyable. Michelle, now 30 years old, was small in stature, very attractive with short dark hair, brown eyes, vivacious personality, and always very warm and friendly. She had many talents, among them being an accomplished pianist. They were both well known in San Jose social circles, highly respected, with many friends in the area and so did not want to experience the publicity of a lawsuit, good or bad. However, as Michelle later related, she was very pragmatic and had a strong desire to know what really caused her blindness. She had her doubts that it was solely from a strep throat.

I greeted Dennis and Michelle as they entered my office. Dennis, tall, athletically trim, good looking, had a somewhat depressed look on his face contrary to his usual cheerful demeanor. He walked in with Michelle's arm on his guiding her to a chair. Michelle appeared as vivacious and attractive as ever with her usual pleasant smile lively greeting me. Her piercing dark brown eyes looked directly at me as I greeted her in return, as though she could clearly see me. She now lived in a totally dark world. Having known Michelle for a good part of my life, I found it very depressing to see her in this state of complete blindness.

At that moment the emotions ran deep in all three of us. Michelle was comfortable talking with me because of our long past friendship, even though she was not used to talking to me as an attorney. After a few casual social exchanges, I asked Michelle, "How are you doing adjusting to your blindness?"

Her story was heart wrenching:

"In the first couple months after I found out I was blind, we contacted California State Rehabilitation for help on how to make adjustments. They sent a social worker to my house once a week for three months to teach me how to handle the physical and environmental aspects of being blind such as folding clothes, cooking in my kitchen, and other household chores. On the social worker's first visit, she spent the first thirty minutes or so telling me about her other clients. She was obviously trying to prepare me for what might further happen in my life so she told me of some spouses who couldn't handle the living conditions with a blind spouse, and therefore got divorced. That really fed into my insecurity and vulnerability. To even consider that I would lose my husband because of my blindness was a traumatic blow.

"She then suggested I should move into the State School for the Blind in Emeryville, California [50 miles north of San Jose]. Mind you, I had just lost my eyesight, I'm very insecure, emotionally helpless in my own home, and this woman proposes that I live and stay in new and strange surroundings like the school for the blind. I'd never been away from home before, never went away to college. I felt upside down and out of it, and they were proposing I live away from my family. But we did visit the place. You have to share a room including the bathroom. The closet and the desk drawers were locked because they said blind people steal from the blind! I'm already very insecure, so there was no way I wanted to be in this situation.

"We can't afford to hire full time care for three children. Fortunately, my mother quit her full-time job and comes to my house five days a week. I'm struggling to survive and maintain my family together. At some point, I realized I had to face up to the reality that my three boys, my husband, and I have survived. Nobody is going to be their mother but me, so I had better figure out how the hell I am going to do this with my blindness."

"Michelle, would you be willing to discuss the details of your medical history with me? Specifically, what lead up to your blindness?"

As she agreed, I immediately jumped to the key question on my mind, "Were you taking oral contraceptives at the time this nightmare began?"

"Yes," she responded.

My interest spiked as my suspicions were confirmed. At that moment, my mind reached back to the lecture on the "Pill" by Dr. Williams. If she had not been on the "Pill," the medical mystery would remain unsolved in my mind. That additional fact, however, justified my now searching in our conversation for medical facts that might causally connect her blindness to the "Pill." I now focused on her medical history for buried facts that might make such a connection true.

"Michelle, describe for me any symptoms you experienced from the time you went on the "Pill" until your immediate illness."

She began to tell her story in acute detail. "I've been on the 'Pill' since 1967 from my OB-GYN, Dr. Gossack. He's been my personal physician since 1962. He prescribed Ortho-Novum, 2 mg, and then six months later he switched me to 1 mg. I remained on that dosage until I got ill."

Dr. Gossack was a highly respected physician in the San Jose area, known as conservative in his practice, who did not prescribe medication or excessive dosages unnecessarily.

She suddenly varied from the subject matter stating emphatically, "I have suspicions about the 'Pill' because they told me not to take it ever again when I was released from the hospital, but I don't want to sue any of my doctors."

I assured her that her doctors were probably as innocent as she was if the "Pill" was the culprit. "Michelle, tell me about your health before you went on the 'Pill.'"

"I was in excellent health and had no serious medical problems, other than occasional sinus type headaches. When I went on the 'Pill', the headaches continued, but increasingly became much more severe, more frequent."

"Where were the headaches localized in your head?" I asked.

"Around my eyes, forehead, eyebrows, and cheekbones, and they were associated with a sensitivity to light."

During the week leading up to her illness, Michelle said she felt great. She did not experience any cold symptoms, chills, fever, or anything unusual. She had no colds or sore throats during the months of January or February. Her menstrual cycle commenced Monday, February 10th, during which she experienced the usual "clammy hands," "little sweaty" and a "little chilled," which was all normal for her. She denied shaking chills, sore throat, nor any other cold symptoms occurred.

"Did anything more occur out of the ordinary?"

"While washing dishes, I poked my ring finger at the cuticle with a steak knife. But a couple days later, on Friday evening [February 14, 1969], I went bowling with my best friend, Alice, and felt fine. I even used my cut finger bowling without any pain or problems. When I woke up the next morning, I felt great, got up, dressed, fed my children and went off to pick up Alice to go furniture shopping."

"Were you taking oral contraceptives as instructed at that time?"

"My prescription had run out a day earlier, so I stopped at Gemco pharmacy to pick up a renewal prescription of Ortho-Novum. I took one pill about noon." [1]

"When did major symptoms occur, if at all?"

Michelle explained that afternoon while shopping, she had an onset of a headache, but no other symptoms. She said later that evening while visiting her mother, "The headache became severe.

"I returned home and took two Excedrin for my headache, and since I had missed taking my 'Pill' the day before, I took *a second pill about 9 p.m.* Dr. Gossack told me that if I missed taking a pill on any particular day, I was to take two pills the next day. And then I went to bed." Ortho's patient booklet advised exactly the same as well as Ortho's package insert instructions to the prescribing physician.

Michelle continued. "The headache got worse and I hardly slept that night. Early Sunday morning I woke Dennis up to take my temperature. It was normal."

"Did you call your doctor during the time of these symptoms?

"Yes, that morning," she acknowledged. "Dr. Gossack prescribed medication for my headache, but it didn't help at all. It got even worse, so bad that I called Dr. Gossack again for help. He told me to come to his office even though it was a Sunday. We got there around 2 p.m. that afternoon."

---

1   Gemco was a subsidiary of Lucky Stores. Ortho-Novum was manufactured by Ortho Pharmaceuticals, a wholly owned subsidiary of Johnson & Johnson.

"Did he examine you?"

"Yes, he gave me a thorough examination. During the exam, I was becoming less and less alert, losing awareness of where I was and people around me."

As Michelle was telling her story, Dennis jumped in, "She was really out of it, I was becoming really worried."

Michelle went on, "I complained to Dr. Gossack that sunlight was hurting my eyes. It was totally blinding as though someone had placed my head under a searchlight. I told him I had to keep my eyes closed all the way to his office. Dr. Gossack took my temperature and commented he was surprised it was normal. As he looked into my throat, he said it looked fine and couldn't see any sign of infection anywhere."

This specific description from Michelle and Dr. Gossack was crucial to my suspicions. I thought to myself, if her blindness was the result of a strep throat, as she was evidently and ultimately informed by her other treating physicians, why no early symptoms of infection? What was the basis of their diagnosis?

Michelle stated that Dr. Gossack was, himself, mystified that the only finding he could see or feel was tenderness in the left jugular vein area of her neck. She explained that she thought it was a strain from bowling Friday. The only symptom was a "tremendous terrible headache." He sent her home with stronger pain medication for her headache and advised her to try to get some sleep.

"Did the medication help?" I asked.

"I tried to sleep but couldn't, even with the stronger medication."

"Did any additional symptoms subsequently occur and, if so, when?" I asked.

"Around 6 p.m. that evening my left eye and entire left side of my face began to swell and my headache got even worse."

Dennis interjected. "When I saw the swelling, I decided to call Dr. Gossack again. He told me to take her immediately to O'Connor Hospital emergency."

En route to the hospital, Dennis described how they were both silent with fear trying to understand what was going on.

"We were really scared!"

Michelle had great difficulty describing what occurred during her hospitalization for the obvious reason; she had become very ill. Dennis attempted to fill in with what details he knew but it was very incomplete. He described how her eye and face had swollen badly and she was fading in and out of consciousness. The only information he could obtain from the doctors that evening was that they, too, were mystified as to what was really going on with her. Michelle did say that physicians later told her she almost died that evening in ICU.

"I remember being out of it, hearing people talking around me . . . had this awareness of people praying. I thought, oh my God, I am getting the last rites, I must be really sick. I remember Dr. Sogg [treating neuro-ophthalmologist] coming in to talk to me, I think it was the next day. I recognized then that I couldn't see as he was asking me questions about my vision. It was the first time I realized that I couldn't see. I told him I couldn't see anything, just a bright light is the last thing I remember. I don't remember him saying that I was permanently blind. It was more obscure, like we don't know what's wrong or where it's going. Around that time they finally thought I would make it, at least not die."

⤞

Dr. Finkle, another ophthalmologist, also examined Michelle's eyes around that time and told her that her eyesight was impaired or damaged. Dennis became very concerned and talked with Dr. Finkle himself. He got the impression Dr. Finkle was focused more on other aspects of her illness than her vision. Dennis in his distress was concerned they might overlook entirely the loss of vision.

"When I was being dismissed from the hospital," Michelle continued, "I was talking to Dr. Kosmin [treating hematologist], asking him what do I do about normal living? What can I do and not do? What do I do about birth control? Can I go back on the 'Pill'? Dr. Kosmin told me, 'Absolutely not. You can never take the 'Pill' again because you have a history of blood clots.' After going home and thinking about being blind, a light bulb went on in my head. I can't take those pills now because of blood clots, or it could happen again. Could it have been the cause of my blood clots and blindness? That suspicion is why I was willing to come in and talk to you."

I asked Dennis and Michelle when did they first learn her blindness was permanent?

Michelle said, "I was concerned about it while in the hospital— if it was permanent. But I didn't find out it was permanent until after I left the hospital. Several weeks later, Dr. Sogg, sent me to Stanford Hospital to have a special dye test done. They had me looking into a huge camera looking into my eyes [a venogram/arteriogram]. After the test, Dr. Sogg spoke to Dennis, but said nothing to me and we went home. Later that day, Dennis took me out of the house for a ride. We parked in a parking lot and then he told me *I was permanently blind*! Up to that point I was happy to be home and alive hoping all along that it wasn't permanent."

Dennis expressed the shock and hurt he felt when he was told that Michelle had lost her sight and was completely blind. At this point in our conversation, both Michelle and Dennis became overwhelmed with emotion as their eyes filled with tears.

"Did any of the treating doctors tell you what caused your illness and blindness?" I asked. They both responded that Dr. Sogg and Dr. Lippe had told them it was caused by a strep infection that entered her blood stream probably from a strep throat and her cut finger. With the medical knowledge I had gained over the years, I could not believe this diagnosis.

"I strongly suspect the primary cause of your blindness is blood clotting caused by the birth control pills," I said.

Having heard her nightmare, the progress of her illness, and definite blood clotting events, I felt confident the case at least deserved further investigation.

I asked, "Can I obtain your medical records and review them? I will, of course, need your signed authorization."

I told them about Dr. Williams and his lecture indicating that I would like to call him and also have him review her records. I would then advise them of Dr. Williams' and my opinions before they had to make any decision on whether to pursue any legal action.

They reluctantly agreed, but Michelle warned, "Unless we can be absolutely convinced that the 'Pill' caused my blindness, we will not consent to proceeding with a lawsuit. In no event can we agree to sue any of my physicians involved."

I advised them there was not a lot of time to make a definite decision because the one-year statute of limitations was soon to expire.[2] I explained this deadline would bar them forever from filing a lawsuit. They decided at my urging to retain me on a purely contingent basis to further investigate the case and report back to them my findings. We agreed there would be no cost to them unless we proceeded with litigation and filed a lawsuit, with their consent.

I escorted Michelle and Dennis out of my office and into the reception area asking them to delay the decision on whether to file a lawsuit until they heard back from me. They thanked me for offering to help find an answer.

After the Ahearn's left, I then poked my head into Dick's office where he was busy reviewing documents on another case.

"Dick, I just had the strangest interview of a case with some old friends. Remember that lecture you and I attended by a Dr. Williams who contended the birth control pill caused blood clotting and even blindness?"

"Barely." he responded.

"Well, we may just have such a case," I responded. I gave him the details of Michelle's case, after which he agreed we should look into it further, even though at our own cost of time and money.

I commented, "If there is a case, it will be a shocking one."

---

2   The Statute of Limitations has since been extended to two years for personal injury.

"But keep in mind, Sal," Dick said. "We have the burden of proof. Not only on the issue of causation, but to prove Johnson & Johnson knew it caused blood clotting."

Being the end of the day, and feeling quite depressed, I said goodnight to my partner and left the office. As I got into my car and started my fifteen-minute drive home, I could not escape the very sad, moving story I had just experienced from these old friends.

I pulled into my driveway, anxious to share this sad story with my wife, Laura, who knew Michelle and Dennis well. As I sat at our kitchen table relating some details as she was preparing dinner, Laura suddenly interrupted me.

"Sal, do you remember when I had that episode of wavery vision and ran to see my ophthalmologist, Dr. Banoff? Remember, while examining my eyes, he asked me if I was on the oral contraceptive? I explained to him that my OB-GYN had recently placed me on the 'Pill' for a short time to help regulate my period. Dr. Banoff told me to get off the 'Pill' immediately. He explained that in his examination he was seeing suspicious changes in the vessels of my retina which he thought explained my sudden strange visual problem."

Chapter 2
A Search For The Mysterious Cause

The next morning as I drove to my office, I mapped out in my mind what I needed to do to get an answer as to whether there was a case for Michelle or not. Walking into my office greeting my secretary Betty as I passed her desk, I said, "I left on your desk last night, the medical consent forms from Michelle Ahearn who I interviewed yesterday. I need you to immediately send out the request for her medical records from both her treating physician, Dr. Gossack and O'Connor Hospital. Also, I need the phone number for a Dr. Harold Williams in the Michaud Law Firm in Wichita, Kansas, thanks."

I settled into my office addressing urgent matters on other cases. Betty shortly entered my office handing me the phone number and I immediately placed a call to Dr. Williams, hoping he would be there.

I was lucky and the receptionist was able to connect me to him.

"Dr. Williams, this is Sal Liccardo in San Jose, California. I met you a few months ago at a lecture you gave here in San Jose on the birth control pill. Coincidentally, yesterday I interviewed a client who was on the 'Pill' and suffered total bilateral permanent blindness and I remembered you mentioning blindness as one of the possible consequences of the 'Pill.' Could I retain you to review her medical records and render me your opinion as to whether you think this might be a legitimate "Pill" case?"

We then discussed some of the essential details of Michelle's case, particularly certain medical signs and symptoms she had related to me. He graciously agreed to review the case saying, "I look forward to the receipt of her medical charts and will contact you after my review."

As I hung up the phone, I finished up with some other urgent matters on my desk, grabbed my jacket as I walked past Betty's desk, and said, "Betty, I'll be gone the rest of the day, I'll be buried in medical research at the library of Stanford Medical School."

I felt a sense of urgency to locate some firm evidence, one way or the other, before spending too much time and money on the case. The statute of limitations was constantly looming in my mind, limiting my time in making such a decision.

I entered the majestic Stanford library, found a comfortable location and began my search for the truth. As I poured through the card catalog for any medical writings on the oral contraceptive, I was somewhat surprised at how few references there were. I could find little discussing significant adverse reactions until I stumbled upon a recent British study that appeared quite powerful to me, *Epidemiological and Public Health Aspects of Oral Contraceptives and Thromboembolic Disease*, by Martin Vessey.

My eyes opened wide as I reviewed this study that strongly suggested some possible link between the oral contraceptive, specifically the estrogen component, ethinyl estradiol, and blood clotting disorders. As I digested this content, I realized Dr. Williams' own small personal study was corroborated by this major study in Great Britain. I realized now I would not be wasting my time in pursuing this case.

⁂

It took the usual several weeks to receive Michelle's medical records from the hospital, but Dr. Gossack's office was more forthcoming. As Betty placed his records on my desk, I immediately dug in, anxious to see if they medically confirmed Michelle's story, although I had little doubt.

Dr. Gossack's medical records revealed that on that Sunday office visit he had examined her throat with an examining light, mouth wide open, tongue depressed, which revealed no obstruction, no tonsil inflammation, no edema (swelling), no redness, nor any sign of an infection. His examination of her eyes, fully open at the time, revealed no sign of infection, bulging, edema or inflammation. Her jaws also were negative as to signs of infection, inflammation, or swelling. The glands and lymph nodes in her neck, which are usually involved with an inflammatory process of the throat, were neither inflamed nor enlarged. Her neck was not rigid and no symptom of meningitis existed. He could not hear rales or any sign of respiratory infection.

All that evidence indicated that her illness did not start with an infection, and particularly not with a strep throat, contrary to her treating doctors' explanation to her as she left the hospital. Again, the question that arose in my mind was why did the doctors tell her this?

Later when the voluminous hospital records arrived, I set aside a full weekend at the office to dig in. I hated giving up family time, with five young children at home, but there was little choice as timing was crucial.

I began the review on a Saturday morning. The records confirmed Michelle arrived at O'Connor Hospital at 7:20 p.m., Sunday, February 16th, and was seen by a neurosurgeon, Dr. Lippe, a respected physician by the medical community. He requested lab studies immediately which later came back indicating a strep infection in Michelle's blood stream. This was the first sign of infection anywhere. The records reflected that Dr. Lippe requested a further examination by a hematologist, Dr. Kosmin, because of this blood infection. Dr. Kosmin, after examining Michelle, indicated he also suspected a blood clotting disorder, in *addition* to the strep infection although strep, itself, is known to cause *some* blood clotting.

The first indication of fever in the medical records was about 7:20 p.m. Sunday, February 16th, on admission to Emergency with a temperature of 99.8 degrees. I thought that's too late for infection to have been the cause of this critical illness in that fever should have been one of the earlier symptoms. At 9:00 p.m. Michelle was admitted to a room with temperature of 99 degrees. Blood cultures that were taken were subsequently deemed to be *positive for streptococcus* (strep infection), however, *cultures of the eye and throat were negative*. This was the first indication of *any* infection, but only in the blood stream. At 10 p.m. massive doses of antibiotics were started intravenously and continued for several days. By midnight, extreme edema engulfed her entire face, with bilateral proptosis (bulging eyes) and a soaring temperature to 104 degrees. She was then transferred to the ICU ward, and by 10 a.m. Monday morning, the 17th, she was placed on the critical list.

The question that arose in my mind was how did the infection get into her blood stream and why did it not go anywhere else? As I read on, it appeared the treating doctors had the same question. In a search for a source of infection, at 12:10 p.m., Dr. Brooks performed an exploration of the nose, throat and sinus, under anesthesia, but no infection site could be found. *No source of infection was ever found.*

Sadly, I noted Michelle was not started on anticoagulants (medication to dissolve blood clots) until 1:15 p.m., eighteen hours after she had been admitted. Throughout her hospitalization she exhibited a tender palpable chord in her neck diagnosed by the treating hematologist as a thrombosed jugular vein, and an indurated area of her left cheek, hard "like a walnut" due to thrombosis of the pterygoid plexis (a bundle of tiny veins in the cheek area that connects to the cavernous sinus). It appeared strange to me that different treating doctors were identifying different areas of thrombosis.

While she was hospitalized, the records reflected other physicians were called in to consult, examine, and evaluate Michelle. The ophthalmologist, Dr. Finkel, and an ear, nose and throat specialist, Dr. Brooks, diagnosed Michelle as having a *cavernous sinus thrombosis* (blood clotting of veins behind the nose), and all the other treating doctors considered that a possibility, including her consulting neuro-ophthalmologist, Dr. Sogg. Upon reading this, I said to myself, "Bingo." A cavernous sinus thrombosis, itself, is a severe blood clotting disorder that not only can cause blindness, but almost immediate death.

By morning of the 18th, several hours following anticoagulant therapy, Michelle's temperature dropped and the edema began to subside, however ophthalmic examination of her eyes indicated total bilateral (both eyes) blindness. This observation from the records confirmed to me that the major illness was a blood clotting event since only anticoagulation therapy is what made a difference, and antibiotics did not. Two weeks later a venogram (radiological view of the veins) and arteriogram (view of the arteries) confirmed residual occlusions (clots) in the orbital veins of the left eye, despite a sufficient lapse of time for the clots to have dissolved.

Michelle remained in ICU until February 24th. She was hospitalized for a total of twenty days during which time the attending physicians were still trying to figure out what caused her illness and subsequent blindness, or was it caused solely by a strep infection? She was released from the hospital having recovered from all symptoms, including the strep infection in her blood, but not the blindness. It was permanent.

At discharge on March 9, 1969 she was given a strange triple diagnosis:

1. beta hemolytic streptococcal cellulitis and bacteremia and probable meningitis,

2. bilateral blindness, probably secondary to optic nerve compression and inflammation,

3. orbital vein occlusion, probably bilaterally.

All of which simply meant that she was diagnosed with a strep infection in her blood, which in turn they believed caused inflammation, compression, and extensive swelling of her eyes and face. The strep and consequent swelling caused blood clotting of the veins in the cavernous sinus backing up blood drainage from the optic nerves on both sides resulting in death of the optic nerves, i.e., permanent complete bilateral blindness. In short, a strep infection which they thought probably started in the throat was the sole culprit.

I found it astounding that Michelle's hospital records did not indicate a single reference to her being asked if she had been on the "Pill." These records, of course, would not have contained the records of Dr. Gossack, indicating his prescribing Ortho-Novum for Michelle. I would have thought she and/or Dennis would have been asked at the time of her entry what medications was she taking? Because of the emergency situation she first presented on admission, I assumed they just never got to that issue, or the "Pill" was not specifically mentioned since it's not a usual medication used to treat a disease. But why wasn't she asked over the remaining 20 days she was there? The answer, I guessed, was that such an omission would not have been surprising. No one considered the oral contraceptive as causing anything at that time. Obviously, these treating doctors were not aware of the recent British study.

∽

After the long weekend of being buried in Michelle's medical records, I returned to my office on Monday morning anxious to discuss my conclusions with Dick.

"Dick, do you have a minute? I'd like to tell you what I found in Michelle's records," I said as I entered Dick's office.

"I'm anxious to know," he said.

"They basically confirm, medically, the story that Dennis and Michelle relayed, but most crucial to me is that they confirmed she suffered extensive thrombosis and the source of the strep infection was never located. Neither in her throat, eyes or anywhere else. If we can prove to a jury that the 'Pill' causes thrombosis and, further, that the manufacturer knew this, I believe we have a case."

Dick then expressed some nervousness at my quick conclusion realizing this would be one huge expensive product liability case, costly in time and money.

"I think this is a tough, risky case, Sal."

I wandered back to my office pondering some crucial questions. I had never handled a case against a pharmaceutical manufacturer before, let alone taking on the largest in the world. Because Ortho Pharmaceutical Company, who manufactured Ortho-Novum, was a wholly owned subsidiary of Johnson & Johnson, I would have to include this 130-year-old parent company, known and respected by every American for its band aids, baby powder and baby shampoos, as the primary Defendant in the case. No juror could possibly hold any bias against this giant corporation that entered the daily lives of every American with its popular and needed products. Johnson & Johnson, at this time, was akin to motherhood and apple pie in the minds of the average American. Suing them would lead to an unfavorable "David versus Goliath" situation.

I gave much thought to my leading such litigation. I had entered practice only seven years earlier. My first three years of trial experience were spent defending criminally charged defendants by court appointment, before the existence of a Public Defender's office in Santa Clara County. My first personal injury trial was in late 1963. My first product liability trial was against General

Motors in 1964 alleging a design defect in the Corvair automobile, but I wisely associated a more experienced trial lawyer in that case, David Harney, who really did all the actual trial work while I merely "second chaired" with him. I had tried many major and minor personal injury cases since that time, but never a case as complex, costly and difficult as a prescription drug pharmaceutical trial. I had to ask myself, was I ready to take this on? Was my firm large enough and financially stable enough to see the case not only through trial, but possibly appeal? All these issues were not only disturbing to Dick, but to me as well. Shortly I would have to face these issues if the evidence of the "Pill" involvement in causation proved to exist.

My thought process then shifted from the potential magnitude of this case, to the importance to society if the "Pill" was causing these catastrophic injuries and deaths to thousands of innocent young women throughout the world. This risk could even extend to my own wife and daughters sometime in the future. This was a challenge I could not ignore.

CHAPTER 3
THE STORY UNFOLDS

As the medical records reached our office, Betty immediately forwarded them to Harold Williams. Within a few days I received a call from Harold, "I've reviewed the records, Sal, and I think you have a case. It's clear to me from the records that thrombosis, and not infection, was the major player in this situation. Strep may have played some small role in her ultimate blindness, but the 'Pill' was a major substantial factor in my judgment."

Harold used the term a *substantial factor* in its legal technical interpretation. "Substantial factor" is the legal requirement under California law to prove causation in a court of law. It simply means "more likely than not" or "more probable" to be the cause. Ortho Pharmaceutical Corporation, as the manufacturer, would then be primarily responsible for the failure to provide adequate warnings of *causation of thrombosis* (blood clotting) to doctors and women as a risk of taking their product, the "Pill." There still remained unanswered the vital legal question, "Was this causal relationship known or should it have been known to Ortho?" To find that answer we would have to do extensive discovery and review all the documents on the "Pill" in the hands of Ortho.

I responded to Harold, "Would you be willing to work with me, if I proceed with the case? I could pay you for your time or, alternatively, I would like to associate you as attorney of record with me so that we could work as a team."

"I would probably prefer to associate if that's acceptable with you," Harold replied. The case will require a lot of work and a lot of my time as well so I believe an association would be more practical from each of our perspectives."

We then proceeded to discuss the financial and other aspects of association and I agreed to forward him the necessary association agreement for his signature after receiving the final okay from the clients.

❧

The time had now arrived to obtain a final decision from Michelle and Dennis. I called them and asked if they could meet with me at my office so I could inform them what had occurred since our last meeting. They wasted no time and the very next day, Dennis escorted Michelle into my office.

After the usual greetings, I advised, "I'm concerned because we are at the statute of limitations. It will expire the day after tomorrow. As I previously explained to both of you, we have to file the lawsuit before the one-year from date of injury expires or you will be forever barred. In other words, you will never be able to file a lawsuit after that date. So, the time is here for your final decision. Let me assist you by bringing you up to date on what we've learned.

"Dr. Williams and I have extensively reviewed your medical records and we are both convinced you have a meritorious case, but a difficult one. There was published this very year, a study by the British strongly suggesting an association between the oral contraceptive and blood clotting disorders. Further studies are continuing in Great Britain. Your medical records reveal that the major cause of your illness was blood clotting and not an infection, even though that may have played a minor role. We don't know for sure. In any event, you certainly didn't have a sore throat or any sign of infection anywhere on your body other than what they found in your blood in a simple blood test.

"We assume that Ortho Pharmaceutical Company either knew, or should have known, that blood clotting was a risk of the 'Pill,' but we will never have a certain answer to that until a lawsuit is filed and we obtain a court order requiring Ortho to give us access to their entire records on their studies on the 'Pill.' Proving their knowledge or concealment of such knowledge of the risk is something we have to prove to win the case.

"I've spoken to Harold Williams about associating with me as a lawyer, if you agree to proceed with the case. He indicated he's anxious to do so and obviously strongly believes you have a good case. He's convinced Ortho knew, or certainly should have known if they did the proper studies that the 'Pill' contributes to blood clots."

Dennis and Michelle were still not yet certain they wanted to proceed.

Michelle asked, "Is there some way we can avoid the publicity of filing the case until we have more time to think it through. We're not yet completely on board with you and Dr. Williams. We're not yet convinced that the 'Pill' was the cause of my blindness. We need to see more evidence."

"There is a way I can give you more time to make a decision and avoid the publicity that you fear, but it has some risk. I can file the case in a remote county which would probably escape being noted by our local press. However, I can't guarantee it won't get picked up somehow. That would remove some of the immediate pressure of you having to make a decision now."

Dennis responded, "I think we can take that risk. We don't want to lose our rights to file."

As I walked them to the door, I said, "I appreciate you both responding so quickly to my request for this decision and I'll proceed to file the case in a remote county. Harold and I will continue to accumulate hopefully enough evidence to provide you the comfort you need to proceed with the litigation." They both thanked me and left the office.

I went right to work drafting the complaint entitled *Michelle and Dennis Ahearn v. Johnson & Johnson, Ortho Pharmaceutical Company and Lucky Stores.* By the time I completed my dictation it was late in the afternoon and I was faced with an unusual situation. Betty, my secretary, was on vacation that week and I had to now have the complaint prepared and in the hands of someone to carry the complaint to another county to get it filed by the next day. Panic was setting in. It was impossible to have the complaint typed and delivered for filing in Solano County before the courts would close that day. Because it was near the end of the workday, I had the further complication of trying to persuade one of the other secretaries in the office to stay late and type it for me.

As the senior partner, I decided to use my pull and started by asking the secretaries of the younger associates, one by one, if they could rescue me from my dilemma as I was without a secretary. Despite explaining the statute of limitations was about to expire, one by one, each refused claiming they were too busy that late in the day. None of them had a real excuse that made sense in light of my urgency.

After exhausting all four of our associate's secretaries, as a last resort, I went to my partner Dick's secretary, Joyce, since Dick was out of the office that day. "Joyce, I hate to bother you with this at this late hour, but I'm in a desperate situation. I have to have this complaint typed and in the hands of someone who can travel to Solano County Superior Court [1½ hour drive from our office] to file by tomorrow or the statute of limitations will have run. All the associates' secretaries have refused my request. I know your workload is heavier than the rest, but I don't know where to turn."

Joyce responded without hesitation, "Absolutely I will get this out for you. I can't believe the others weren't willing to help you in this desperate situation." She went right to work on my complaint, which at that time on a typewriter, with carbon paper, involved a couple hours' worth of work in the best of hands.

While Joyce worked on the complaint, I went back to each of the four secretaries who had refused my desperate plea and told them not to return to work the next day, they would receive a check in the mail for two weeks' pay. I fired them. The foregoing unforgettable event became known in the office and beyond, among the secretarial world, as "Sal's St. Valentine Massacre" at the Caputo, Liccardo office. My thoughts as I left the office that late evening, "What a rough way to start this difficult case, I hope this isn't a bad omen."

◌⁄◌

This strategy of filing in a remote county worked. Under the procedural law at the time, I could transfer the case to Santa Clara County at a later date, the legally proper county in which the case was to be pursued. This procedure allowed the Ahearns more time to decide if they wanted to proceed. This process, of course, would further allow me more time to investigate and research the case.

Over the next couple months, Harold Williams and I continued to search the medical literature for any reported case of bilateral permanent blindness arising from a strep infection. We could not find a single anecdotal case in all of medical history. During one of my many days of being buried in Stanford Medical School Library on this case, I stumbled upon a medical article authored by the head of the department of pharmacology at a major American university medical school.

He was a pharmacologist, M.D., Ph.D., highly respected and recognized worldwide for his expertise particularly in the field of prescription drugs. Although his article did not directly indicate oral contraceptives as a medical risk for blood clotting, it struck me as raising this issue between the lines. It advocated for more research and studies on oral contraceptives as to potential risks associated with their use. He even discussed the British studies and their suggested association with blood clotting but took no firm position.

I took a long shot and contacted him by telephone asking if he would be willing to review Michelle's medical records, and whether I could retain him to render his opinion on the case? When he agreed, I sent him her entire medical record.

A couple of months passed before I received a call from him, rather than the customary medical report. He told me he had completed his review of the medical records, and was ready to discuss the case with me, but he refused to discuss it over the phone. Instead, he asked if we could meet at his office on the campus of the medical school where he was teaching. His follow up was shocking to me, "Come alone. Do not bring anyone with you." In my entire 56 years of active trial practice, I have never experienced such a request from a medical consultant.

When I arrived at his office a few days later, I was immediately escorted by his assistant into his personal office not knowing what to expect. As I entered, he was sitting at his desk, a scholarly looking gentleman appearing to be in his mid-sixties, with stacks of books and medical literature surrounding him. I spotted Michelle's medical chart near him. He graciously greeted me, offered me a seat, and then closed the door. His first question to me was, "What do you want to know?"

I responded immediately. "Does the oral contraceptive cause blood clotting in some women?"

"The reason I asked you to come alone is that if you repeat a single word that I am about to tell you, I will deny it. I risk losing my position as head of the pharmacology department at this school, and possibly even my teaching job. The pharmaceutical industry, including Johnson & Johnson, provides significant financial support to this medical institution and its students in the form of various medical supplies such as stethoscopes, drugs, etc. You will better understand after I answer your question. I believe *the oral contraceptive is the biggest fraud ever perpetuated upon American womanhood."*

Shocked by his powerful response, I asked, "Was the oral contraceptive a substantial factor in causing Michelle's blindness?"

Without hesitation, he responded with a clear, definitive *"Absolutely!"*

I was again shocked by his certainty. This was unusual from a physician consultant. I quickly followed up, "I have a third question," to which he said, "I think I know what that is."

I asked, "Will you testify to your opinion at trial in this case?"

"I thought that would be your next question, and the answer is no for the reasons I have already explained to you, however, I will assist you in finding the experts you need who will testify in your case."

He followed through with his promise and immediately referred me to a superb expert ophthalmologist who was Professor Emeritus at Stanford University Medical School, in Palo Alto, California, Gerald Bettmen, M.D., Ph.D. Dr. Bettmen was also an advisor to the Federal Drug Administration (FDA) on ophthalmological drugs dealing with the eyes and vision.

I contacted Dr. Bettmen and told him that I had been referred specifically to him as someone who might be willing to testify in the *Ahearn* case. I asked him if he would review Michelle's medical records to advise me of his opinions. He contacted me after his first review and invited me to his home to discuss the case. When I arrived, he greeted me warmly, a short studious looking man, appearing to be in his mid or late 70's, wearing unusually thick glasses. Following my usual custom with expert witnesses, I started to assess in my mind whether he would appear appealing and persuasive to a jury in a courtroom conveying a positive impression.

We discussed the case in great detail.

He confirmed, "There is not a single case, either from my medical experience or in the medical literature, of a sore throat caused by a strep infection resulting in total permanent bilateral blindness. I believe the mechanism of Michelle's blindness started with thrombosis in a tiny collection of venous blood vessels located in the area of the cheek bone called the pterygoid plexis. The blood clotting then spread to the veins of the cavernous sinus, clotting the veins draining blood from the optic nerves. This venous backup then caused the arterial blood vessels feeding blood to the optic nerves to thrombose [clot] depriving oxygenated blood to the optic nerves of both eyes. The cells of the optic nerve then died resulting in the blindness."

"Doctor, do you believe there was more than one cause that contributed to her blindness?"

"Yes, there are three factors that played a role in rendering Michelle more at risk to blood clotting. She had a strep infection in her blood, and she had type B blood, each of which synergistically increased her risk of clotting and set her up for the most significant risk factor, the two oral contraceptive pills she took that day. *She was a sitting duck for blood clotting from the oral contraceptive.*"

I asked if he would be willing to testify at trial to that opinion. Without hesitation he enthusiastically agreed.

℘

As I drove back to my office, my thoughts were plentiful. I was now convinced not only that the "Pill" was the primary cause of Michelle's blindness, but I now had a strong persuasive well qualified expert witness to explain with solid medical reasoning, why Michelle went blind. Dr. Bettman's powerful reasoning and persuasiveness removed any doubt in my mind, especially when considered on top of what the eminent pharmacologist had shared with me, that the "Pill" was "the greatest fraud ever perpetuated upon American womanhood." My enthusiasm to proceed with the case exploded. How could any trial lawyer worth his or her salt now shy away from such a potentially powerful case?

I had reached the point where I needed to obtain my clients' consent before progressing any further and incurring any further costs of expert consultation. When I arrived back to my office, I called Michelle and Dennis and told them I had crucial information to share with them so that they could make their final decision.

A few days later, Dennis escorted Michelle into my office, both anxious to hear what I had to say. I told them about being referred to Dr. Bettman, a renowned Ophthalmologist, who was willing to testify with sound reasoning and persuasiveness that the "Pill" was a substantial factor in causing her blindness. I explained that Michelle's blood type, together with taking two pills, convinced Dr. Bettman that she was "a sitting duck" to experience a severe blood clotting event. Michelle's blood type was known to be susceptible to clotting, and not even that fact was referred to in any of the medical information distributed on the "Pill." This made Michelle even more upset and angry at Johnson & Johnson. After hearing from me all of the foregoing, Michelle responded, *"Had I known that risk, I never would have taken it!"*

I then explained to them what a competent scholarly pharmacologist told me, "The 'Pill' is the '. . . biggest fraud ever perpetuated upon American womanhood.'"

Michelle immediately commented. "Biggest fraud on women? They were injuring and killing people and didn't give a damn!"

As Michelle and Dennis digested all this new information, their past lingering doubts about proceeding with litigation completely evaporated. They had now become crusaders for the truth and gave me authority to proceed with the litigation to its end. They no longer doubted that their case was clearly meritorious and their cause was just. Their goal was no longer solely for their own personal benefit, but more to save the lives of unknowing women taking the "Pill."

Now authorized to proceed with the litigation, I discussed with Michele and Dennis the details of a fee agreement. Dennis commented, "We're not wealthy and couldn't possibly pay you and Harold by the hour."

"There's no need to pay us an hourly fee. We can proceed on a contingency basis. If we should lose, you would owe my firm nothing. We will take the entire financial risk of loss. This is the usual fee arrangement in product liability tort cases."

Dennis then requested a modification to the percentage of fee to which I agreed. "If it weren't for this contingent fee arrangement, we could not continue with the litigation." Dennis confirmed.

I further explained, "We would advance all the costs as we have to date and will be reimbursed for such costs from any recovery. If we lose, we will not seek reimbursement of these costs. Your only risk is that if we lose, Johnson & Johnson will have the right to pursue certain defense costs against you."

I gave them a rough estimate of what the range of such costs could be, and this factor did not deter them from wanting to proceed with the lawsuit. I thanked them as I escorted them out of my office, commenting, "My work is now cut out for me, I have much to do."

I called Dr. Gossack to arrange a conference with him. Several days later as I entered his office, I found Dr. Gossack to be courteous and cooperative. The first thing I said to him was, "Doctor, you are not a party in this lawsuit, nor is any physician. We believe you physicians were kept in the dark about the thrombosis risk of the 'Pill,' as were your patients."

I then explained the case solely involved the right of a woman to know the risks of the "Pill" before taking it and the anticipated timeline of the case. I told him that Dr. Bettman, from Stanford, agreed to testify to his opinion that the "Pill" caused Michelle's blindness and explained his reasoning. Dr. Gossack was quite receptive recognizing the specific expertise of Dr. Bettman and acknowledged that he, as an OB-GYN, was not an expert on the risks of the "Pill." Dr. Gossak expressed his honest opinion that he, too, was completely unaware of the risks of the "Pill," and had he known he certainly would have warned Michelle. He recognized that he was not the only physician lacking knowledge of the "Pill's" risk at the time. I discussed with him some recent article in the medical literature which we found indicating that blood type could be a risk factor when combined with the "Pill." He acknowledged he was not aware of that fact and knowing that Michelle had Type B blood, he probably would not have recommended the "Pill" to her at all, if that's true.

The pharmaceutical industry had done a successful job promoting the safety of the "Pill" and concealing these risks from the entire American medical profession. For these reasons, I did not consider for a moment that Michelle's prescribing doctor shared any responsibility for what had happened to her, as I told him so at the time. He, too, was deprived of *the right to know*, so I explained that he was never considered as a possible defendant. He communicated his feeling this litigation could be as helpful to prescribing physicians as to Michelle. I asked if he would cooperate in testifying to a jury on Micelle's medical history and his lack of information on the clotting risks of the "Pill." He did not hesitate to agree to help in any way he could with his knowledge of the case.

At this point I felt that I had a meritorious case well worth pursuing, not only for Michelle and Dennis, but for the millions of American women who were on the "Pill," or would be. Further, the case would provide a service to their respective unknowing prescribing physicians, all having no idea of the risk to which they were exposing their patients.

❧

I returned to my office and prepared the necessary pleadings to transfer the venue of the lawsuit from Solano County to Santa Clara County Superior Court. In addition to Johnson & Johnson and Ortho Pharmaceutical, I had also named in that complaint, Gemco, whose pharmacy sold the oral contraceptive to Michelle and its parent, Lucky Stores. As California entities doing business in Santa Clara County, they provided the diversity of defendant residents required by law to avoid the case being transferred to a

Federal District Court, and then possibly to the East Coast, the home of Ortho and Johnson & Johnson. Gemco and Lucky Stores were in the chain of commerce with Ortho, thereby having a duty, *under the law*, to warn as well, and therefore were a legitimate named party to the lawsuit. Their financial exposure was nil because of an industry custom where a manufacturer, as the primary culprit, would not only defend such retailers, but would indemnify them from any loss.

The lawsuit was based upon the failure of the Defendants to warn of the risks of the "Pill" which caused Michelle's blindness, and not that the "Pill" should never have been placed on the market. The next legal step was to serve the complaint on each of the Defendants. This commenced what was to become a long, complicated, expensive legal battle. Truly, it had become a David vs. Goliath situation!

CHAPTER 4
DIGGING FOR GOLD

Neither Johnson & Johnson nor the other parties were aware they had been sued in that the complaint had not yet been served on them. The time of awakening had now arrived, and I had the complaint setting forth the critical facts of the case finally served on the Defendants. Johnson & Johnson probably was not shocked by the contents in general, having by that time defended and won other cases involving the same product. However, the contents of the complaint identifying bilateral blindness as a consequence of their product, would certainly have been alarming.

Johnson & Johnson retained a law firm to defend them and the other Defendants, out of Sacramento, California, namely Fitzwilliam, Memeering, Stumbos, and DeMers, a well-known defense firm. The firm assigned the case, as their lead counsel, to Marion H. Pothoven, a competent and intelligent trial lawyer, well experienced defending major corporations. He was a pleasant appearing, rather large man with a low baritone voice, very commanding and persuasive in the courtroom. He was also a man of integrity.

Harold and I, together with my past secretary, Betty Edgar, who by this time was a very competent paralegal, constituted the entire team representing Michelle and Dennis in this monstrous case. This was quite tiny contrasted with the army of people working against us.

We were now faced with the complex process of commencing discovery on Ortho and Johnson & Johnson, hoping to find the hard evidence that they knew the blood clotting risk of the "Pill," before it was prescribed to Michelle. A critical value of formal discovery is that all responses whether written or oral are under oath.

We prepared and sent written interrogatories (questions to be answered under oath) to Johnson & Johnson and Ortho. The areas of inquiry ranged from proper identification of entities to the history of the oral contraceptive, including pre-marketing and post-marketing studies.

When their answers came back, they provided us with the location of the New Drug Application (NDA) on their Ortho-Novum pill. Federal Law requires that a pharmaceutical company maintain an NDA containing almost every document initiated and received pertaining to their pharmaceutical product. The NDA would potentially contain a world of knowledge and information on what they knew and did not know at any particular time frame. Further, through this process we were able to identify names of key Ortho people involved with the testing and marketing of Ortho-Novum, as well as the existence and location of key documents. Among those people identified by Ortho was a vice president, who was their medical director and the person most knowledgeable on the entire history of Ortho's involvement with the oral contraceptive. We were sure he would play a major role in this case.

The Defense subpoenaed all of Michelle's medical records and then proceeded to take oral depositions of witnesses, the usual process in a product liability case. They took Michelle's deposition, questioning her on every aspect of her life and her health, including the details of her illness that lead to her blindness. She was excellent in directly answering each question truthfully and convincingly over a two-day period, not an easy task for any witness. The Defense could not intimidate her despite their several attempts. Her story was truthful, emotional and compelling.

Michelle was extensively questioned on her relationship with Dr. Gossack as her OB-GYN. She testified that Dr. Gossack had originally prescribed 2 mg. and then reduced her to 1 mg. And that he never told her about any significant risks to the oral contraceptive, particularly, she was never told by anyone she had the risk of going blind. She stated that on one visit to his office, she saw Ortho-Novum pamphlets displayed on a table next to her, so she picked one up, perused it and took it home with her. She did not see any warnings in the pamphlet about any serious risk or side effects whatsoever.

Dennis likewise did an excellent job in his deposition, again creating a very moving story of their life together, especially handling the daily challenges of her blindness. Most sensible Defendants would want to discuss settlement after these powerful depositions, but not Johnson & Johnson. They, like many other "Pill" manufacturers, were going to fight the case to the end primarily because the odds, based upon the many past defense verdicts, were clearly in their favor.

Thereafter, the Defense pursued the depositions of each of her treating physicians, not only for the illness resulting in her blindness, but covering her entire past medical history, primarily looking for some medical evidence that would support their defense argument that her blood clotting was spontaneous, and not caused by the "Pill."

Michelle's OB-GYN, Dr. Gossack testified in his deposition how he was prescribing the oral contraceptive to his patients following the instructions he had been given by the representative of the pharmaceutical manufacturers and their written handout instructions. He even kept Ortho-Novum pamphlets, provided by Ortho, in his waiting room for his patients to read and take with them. These pamphlets, in fact, described the wonders of this "Pill" that would allow women of childbearing age to avoid or put off pregnancy. It emphasized the "Pill" as "safe" and "natural," and advised a woman that if she should miss a day, she should take two pills the following day to ensure her protection from pregnancy. Nothing was said about the risk of developing thrombosis or blood clots that could result in stroke, heart attacks, paralysis, blindness or death. This was the pamphlet Michelle had read and taken home.

❧

Among the marvelous tools the law provides in the search for the truth, is the right to seek an order from the court requiring access to crucial documentary evidence. In the face of a court order, any attempt to destroy or conceal the requested evidence results in severe sanctions and penalties. A major hurdle for us was to gain access to all the documentary evidence in the hands of Ortho pertaining to every aspect of the development, testing, marketing of the "Pill," and the NDA. This necessitated us to file with the Court a motion to obtain a court order requiring Ortho to provide access to such documents. Ortho did not want us to have access to their entire NDA so seeking that order was our first major battleground.

I filed the motion in the Superior Court of Santa Clara County requesting the Court to order Ortho to provide us access to their entire NDA, and all documents pertaining to their research, pre-marketing and post-marketing testing, studies, and the like. Ortho filed extensive opposition to our motion contending such an order would violate privileged trade secrets and involve an excessive burden in time and cost to provide access and therefore constitute extreme harassment. They argued the documents, constituting the entire NDA, were in the hundreds of thousands thereby imposing extensive time burdens on Ortho's people to just pull together and organize them for such an inspection. The costs, they argued would also be prohibitive, and at the least should be borne by the Plaintiffs.

A hearing occurred involving extensive oral argument from both sides. The Court rejected most of their arguments, except for their request some documents be kept confidential up to the time of trial, thereby granting the order.

After obtaining the order, I called Harold in Wichita advising him that we were successful—he was ecstatic. He explained that in other cases against Ortho around the country, no plaintiff was yet able to obtain a court order as broad as this, i.e., to view and copy their entire NDA. Consequently, we nor anyone else in the litigation had any advance knowledge of what the contents might be, except of course Ortho and possibly the FDA.

I was grateful to the wisdom of this local Judge in refusing to allow Ortho to limit what they made available for our inspection, implicitly recognizing the corporate temptation to conceal critical documents. Included in the order was the right to review and copy all communications from any source pertaining to the "Pill."

⁕

In subsequent days Harold and I had many discussions on how we might take advantage of this great order. I asked Harold, "You've seen these NDAs from other pharmaceutical companies, what are we dealing with in terms of volume and time in our search for useful evidence for trial?"

"You and I need to go to Raritan and be prepared to spend several weeks, if necessary, searching for the evidence we need to properly review them. My wife, Betty, would also be helpful in that she's familiar with the NDA documents as well." We discussed the timing for the trip. I would fly nonstop to Philadelphia where we would meet, obtain portable copying equipment and then proceed to Raritan, New Jersey, Ortho's headquarters where all their records were housed.

With Court Order in hand, I climbed aboard my transcontinental flight for a potential three-week trip. As I looked down at the clouds thinking about spending weeks away from my family reviewing documents, this quickly became a trip I dreaded. Arriving in Philadelphia late that evening, I met up with Harold and Betty at a downtown restaurant where we chatted over dinner on what to anticipate.

Early the next morning, with the portable mimeograph machine in the trunk of our rental car, we drove to Raritan and checked into a local hotel, our new home away from home, had some breakfast and then drove to Ortho's headquarters. Arriving at 9 a.m., we were led into a small approximately 12' by 12' interior room with only a small table and a couple of chairs. There were no windows and only one door, a claustrophobic and uncomfortable work area. An employee of Ortho was guarding that door as we were led into the room. His presence was obviously to observe everything we did and hear every word we said among ourselves.

After waiting about 30 minutes, a cart with 4 levels of shelves was wheeled into the room. It was loaded with binders containing their NDA and other "Pill" related documents. Under the watchful eye of Ortho, we each began to pull a binder off the cart and commence our review. As we would spot a document of interest and presumable evidentiary value, we would hand it to Betty to copy. Strangely, the Ortho guard failed to question or record any history of the specific documents we were copying. He just stood there obviously straining to listen to anything we said.

In short, we were not allowed any privacy to discuss the contents of any document, or whether it deserved to be copied without being overheard by Ortho's people. Harold and I, realizing the situation, stepped out of the room for a moment feigning to need a restroom, and quickly created a speaking code of sorts between us to use when we spotted a document that was important evidence and therefore needed to be copied. Harold suggested we should not describe, with any specificity, any key document, but rather verbally downplay its importance as we handed them to Betty to copy.

As we began our review, we quickly noticed that many of these documents neatly contained in binders were intentionally internally disorganized and scrambled! Page three of a document would be without pages one and two. These missing pages would later appear on another day on another cart. Even the subject matter lacked continuity within the binders on a particular cart, as well as from cart to cart, day to day. Ortho had done everything possible to burden and frustrate our discovery. That, of course, rendered our job incredibly difficult and time consuming beyond the normal. Imagine the cost to Ortho to process this deliberate scramble of documents and later put it back together. That, no doubt, was on Ortho's mind when they argued to the judge that it would be too burdensome to produce these documents.

Despite these intentionally obstructional and frustrating tactics imposed by Ortho, our efforts immensely payed off. In the world of evidence, we struck gold! We discovered overwhelming documentation of a deliberately designed cover-up of serious side effects at their pre-marketing testing level. Ortho would deliberately select physicians as study directors who would bias their studies by using clinics located among an uneducated, poor, transit population of women that would most likely *never return to the clinic if they developed serious side effects*. Rather, such patient would entirely disappear or drop out from the study. Most likely they could have ended up in some public hospital or morgue. The study records merely labeled them as "no shows" if they did not show up for the next monthly prescription of pills. No effort would be made to follow up as to why that particular woman no longer came to the clinic. Due to the very nature and demographics of the clinic population, it would be impossible to follow up on most of the drop out patients. The question would remain as we reviewed these studies, "Was she a drop out because she moved, became ill from the 'Pill,' or died from the 'Pill'?" The lack of follow up greatly discredited the epidemiological reliability of the reported outcome of the majority of these clinical studies used by Ortho to argue that thrombosis was not a risk.

⌒

As we waded through thousands of documents, I stumbled upon more gold. I handed a document to Harold, commenting, "Is this really worth copying?"

Harold paused for a moment as he quickly read the document and he responded quietly, "It's probably not worth copying, I don't know, Sal."

"What the hell, Betty, go ahead and copy it," I said.

The document was addressed from a prominent physician from upstate New York who wrote to Dr. Arnold Cronk, vice-president and medical director of Ortho, offering his clinic as an ideal location for clinical studies on the "Pill." He described his patient population as well educated, middle class women whose medical history would be well known to the clinic because of having been patients of the clinic for many years. This physician emphasized that because of the forgoing, any pre-existing medical problems would be well known, and any occurrence of new side effects would thereby be easier to detect. A further advantage he pointed out was that there would be *no loss of follow-up* because their patients lived in the same location for many years. Dr. Cronk's reply letter in a nutshell was a crisp, "No thank you, doctor."

Harold later stumbled upon another gold nugget. He handed me page 2 of a 3-page letter, and mumbled, "Is this worth copying? I don't think so." which became our code to copy.

I looked at it and said calmly, "Probably not Harold, but throw it on the copier for the hell of it." The guard at the door seemed to have a puzzled look at our remarks.

Neither of us could barely hold back our glee. A Dr. Goldzhier, an endocrinologist, with a clinic in El Paso, Texas, on the border of Mexico, wrote this letter to Dr. Cronk also soliciting Ortho's selection of his clinic for testing the "Pill." He described his clinic population as ideal for a pre-marketing study noting that his clinic patient population was: "... *uneducated, illiterate, and mostly Mexican and white trash* who would not recognize nor report side effects," from the "Pill" being tested on them. Dr. Cronk responded quickly, accepting his offer and retained him as Ortho's major pre-marketing clinical investigator on the safety of the "Pill."

As we left for our hotel that day, we could not hold back our excitement over finding such powerful material evidence that would certainly have a favorable impact on a jury.

As we continued our days of discovery, among the thousands of documents produced by Ortho we found over 300 adverse reaction reports by individual doctors concerning their observations in their own patients. The earliest of such reports went back to 1962, shortly after the "Pill" was first approved by the FDA. One such report dated in 1966 was from a Dr. Harris, with a specialty in internal medicine, practicing at the time in Mt. View, California, 10 miles north of San Jose. Harold pulled this together then handed it to me to review. When I saw the first page of this document, I was not so impressed, but as Harold handed me further pages, including additional correspondence between the parties, I recognized that this was really powerful evidence of causation. I looked at Harold and said, "This is an awful lot of pages to copy, I'm not sure it's worth it."

"You're probably right, but Betty started copying the first few pages, we might as well finish."

In this series of documents, Dr. Harris described his patient as having no prior history of thrombosis or phlebitis but developed thrombophlebitis (blood clotting in the legs) after being prescribed the "Pill." She was a mother of six children. He took her off the "Pill," treated her thrombophlebitis, and she recovered. He wrote to Dr. Cronk asking if there was any information linking the "Pill" to thrombosis? Dr. Cronk replied there was absolutely no evidence of a link between the "Pill" and thrombophlebitis or blood clotting, and that his patient probably had a past history of the disease.

Relying on the advice of the medical director and vice president of Ortho, Dr. Harris put his patient back onto the "Pill." She developed thrombophlebitis for a second time. He immediately took her off the "Pill," and treated the thrombophlebitis until she again recovered. Dr. Harris then wrote a second letter to Dr. Cronk explaining what had happened a second time. Dr. Cronk replied with the same contention that there was no evidence it caused blood clotting in any form. He again advised that the "Pill" was absolutely safe.

Dr. Harris believed Dr. Cronk and placed his patient on the "Pill" a *third time*. This time his patient developed a pulmonary embolism (a blood clot that migrates) in the pulmonary artery of the lungs, which if not immediately treated is fatal. With immediate hospital emergency treatment, she recovered. Dr. Harris wrote back a scathing letter to Dr. Cronk telling him what had happened *a third time.* She was taken off the "Pill" and had no further episodes of any blood clotting disease.

As we left Ortho's headquarters that day and were finally free to converse, we almost jumped for joy at the finding of this classic triple "challenge and response" situation right within the records of the Defendant. A "challenge and response" describes an event where a patient is challenged with a particular drug and shortly thereafter develops certain side effects to that drug. When the drug is withdrawn, the patient recovers. When challenged a second time, the patient develops the same side effect again. When the drug is again withdrawn recovery occurs. In medical science this is powerful evidence of a cause and effect relationship between the specific drug and the specific side effect. To some medical scientists, a challenge and response situation carries more weight as evidence of *cause and effect* than an epidemiological study, whether retrospective or prospective. Dr. Harris' letters described for Ortho a triple challenge and response that left little opportunity of it occurring by mere chance.

"Harold, somehow this has to be our first evidence introduced to the jury. No jury is going to believe Ortho did not know they had this problem with this kind of evidence in their own hands."

Harold agreed, "Sal, how are we going to introduce this evidence without Dr. Cronk on the stand which won't be till near the end of the trial?"

"I'll find a way," I replied.

Overall, we discovered a total of six challenge and response case reports in Ortho's records in Raritan. This discovery process went on for more than two weeks, before I had to return to California to handle the many motions Ortho was continuously filing to obstruct our discovery rights. Harold and his very capable wife, Betty, continued the documentary review process in Raritan for an additional week and a half.

Among Ortho's records of over 300 adverse case reports, they included 5 cases of blindness, a few cases of optic neuritis, vascular occlusions (blood clots) in and about the eyes and *50 death cases*, all prior to Michelle's blindness. In many cases thrombosis was reported as occurring in unique sites such as the intestine, kidney, auxiliary vein in the arm, abdominal veins, and other unusual areas where thrombosis was not known to occur spontaneously.

On my flight home, I thought to myself, what powerful evidence these challenge and response cases contributed to the issue of causation which we had to prove. I especially dwelled on the triple challenge and response of Dr. Harris and how I could make this the first evidence seen by the jury at trial.

I couldn't help wondering why Ortho did not warn physicians or patients of a potential causation between the "Pill" and thrombosis, or at least tell them about Dr. Harris's triple challenge and response if there was any integrity in the company. In follow-up interrogatories on Ortho, we learned that these challenge and response case reports received by Ortho were *never reported to the FDA*. I wondered at the fact that Dr. Harris' triple challenge and response was reported to Dr. Cronk at Ortho three years before Michelle's catastrophic event, well within sufficient time to have provided a warning to Dr. Gossack and Michelle if made known. That fact rendered the reported triple challenge and response as certainly relevant to Michelle's case. Harold and I added this evidence to our pot of gold uncovered in Raritan, New Jersey.

Arriving back and returning to work, I called Michelle and Dennis asking if they would come to my office so I could bring them up to date on the evidence we discovered. As I described the manner in which Ortho deliberately manipulated their pre-market and post-market studies to reduce the reporting of side effects, particularly, thrombosis, Michelle became very upset.

She exclaimed, "It's horrible that a well-known and respected pharmaceutical giant like Johnson & Johnson would phony-up their studies and ignore case reports. This makes me feel more positive about my lawsuit, learning that Big Pharma is deliberately and systematically hurting women, and they don't care—it's all for profit. This is a big reason for me suing. I need to let women know!"

In the ensuing two years of trial preparation, many depositions were taken of physicians involved in the treatment of Michelle, followed by depositions of designated experts identified by each side. All during this time, not only did Harold and I continue our search of the medical literature for positive evidence of causation and notice to the pharmaceutical manufacturers, but we were still searching to find a single case of bilateral blindness from a strep throat. We also used the opportunity of time to accumulate the ongoing depositions and document discovery that was being pursued in the many other "Pill" cases pending within the United States. There was ongoing cooperation among all the plaintiff lawyers handling these cases which reduced somewhat the need to do all the litigation discovery in our case. An answer under oath, in one case, can be used in another case so long as the issues are similarly relevant.

However, a significant area of discovery remained to be explored. What did Ortho's detail men know and what did they tell physicians about the "Pill?" The pharmaceutical industry uses representatives called a "detail man" to personally call upon physicians to tout their drugs. This is the only real direct contact a doctor has with a manufacturer and such was the case with the "Pill." A physician expects the detail man to honestly convey the most recent information on their product, i.e., effective dosage use, precautions on use, side effects, latest studies, and the most recent findings. Was this the practice of Ortho's detail men?

To get the answer to this question, my wife, Laura, and I traveled to Puerto Rico in early 1974 to take the deposition of Ortho's detail man, Thomas Preston. Thomas Preston called upon Dr. Gossack from 1965 through March 1969. In 1974, he was still working for Ortho in San Juan, Puerto Rico.

Mr. Preston testified that when he would call upon Dr. Gossack, he would emphasize the value of the "Pill" as a contraceptive, but *never* discussed adverse effects other than what was contained in the package insert or patient booklets. He stated that Ortho never requested its detail men to solicit adverse reaction reports, to convey information on adverse reaction reports received, nor to discuss the relationship between the "Pill" and thrombosis in any manner with the physician. He confirmed that this was never done with Dr. Gossack as well. His testimony confirmed the lack of warning by Ortho, not only to Michelle's treating OB-GYN, but to doctors generally throughout the United States as of the late 1960's.

Thus, the power of discovery and court orders dug hard evidence out of Big Pharma's dungeon that brought the truth to light.

CHAPTER 5
A BLACK CLOUD ON THE HORIZON

Fear of losing the *Ahearn* case hovered like a black cloud over the tremendous effort and monetary case costs that were soaring daily. The case was set to commence trial on October 28, 1974. By early 1974, so many "Pill" cases had already proceeded to trial throughout the United States with wins for the various pharmaceutical manufacturers, that fear among those of us awaiting trial grew by leaps and bounds. The many consistent losses foretold a dismal future for this litigation nationwide.

Every law firm involved in these cases asked the same questions: Can the pharmaceutical industry be beat in a court of law? Can a jury be convinced of their wrongdoing in concealing the truth from doctors and the public about the horrendous risks of the "Pill?" And if so, how? The industry spared no expense or effort to defeat the plaintiff in every case. They used every resource available to them and it was working. Most importantly, they had public opinion on their side.

The popularity of the "Pill" to doctors and the public at large was overwhelming by 1974. After all, the "Pill" was saving the world. Not the least, was that it provided an easy and "safe" option to pregnancy, and to many, a much wiser choice than abortion. Who would want to believe that this easy perfect birth control solution might be dangerous? Who would keep an open mind to any argument that the "Pill" was bad? Therefore, the public mindset was for the continuation of the "Pill" and not its demise, nor restrictive use. People of this thinking would be the prospective jurors who would decide these future cases. How could we possibly convince any prospective juror that the "Pill" was so dangerous when their bias was to believe it had to be safe. How could we possibly win?

Trial lawyers handling these cases recognized this public biased mindset, and the proven expertise of the pharmaceutical industry's success in its ability to prey upon this bias. One of these trials lawyers was Paul Rheingold, respected in the field of pharmaceutical litigation. Paul was a close friend to Harold Williams and had originally joined us in the *Ahearn* case agreeing to share in the risks for a percentage of the outcome. However, about this time, Paul recognizing all the forgoing negative factors, called and asked if he could withdraw from the case. He expressed his opinion that we had no real chance of success. Appreciating the effect of this black cloud of fear harboring over many lawyers in this litigation, I had no problem understanding his desire to withdraw, so I agreed. I did somewhat arrogantly state to Paul that we had powerful evidence from discovery that made our case different from those already tried, and therefore I thought he was making a mistake. He stuck to his decision to withdraw.

During this trial preparation phase, I had the opportunity to observe many days of a trial in Northern California against Searle for causing a stroke to a woman on their "Pill." The artificial estrogen component, ethinyl estradiol, was the same as in Ortho's. In fact, because of this similarity, we learned during our discovery of Ortho's documents, Ortho and Searle had entered into an agreement during pre-marketing testing to exchange adverse reaction reports. That agreement allowed each to know what adverse reactions ethinyl estradiol was causing. Interestingly, there was no evidence this agreement was ever disclosed to the FDA.

This Searle case was tried by another brilliant trial lawyer, Paul Melodia, of the Walkup firm in San Francisco. Paul and I had worked together for a couple of years in the preparation of each of our cases, exchanging discovery, deposition transcripts, ideas, and strategies. Despite Paul doing an excellent job trying the case, he too could not break through that "Pill" bias in the jury's mind. Thus, another win for the pharmaceutical industry and a loss for the injured woman.

As Harold and I spent much time analyzing the various risks in the cases, and the litigation history, Harold came up with an invaluable concept. We plaintiff trial lawyers should all get together for a three-day seminar to brainstorm with one another on how to beat Big Pharma. Harold suggested that he get his senior partner in his Wichita, Kansas firm to host the event since it would be located in the middle of the country more accessible for lawyers nationwide. The firm had almost 100 pending "Pill" cases at the time awaiting trial.

Harold and the senior partner of his firm, a great mid-western trial lawyer, Gerald (Gerry) Michaud, agreed to host the seminar on a weekend in mid-January. Though somewhat convenient to many, being roughly mid-distance from both coasts, its January temperature of zero degrees F. was not so inviting. Yet many attended. Gerry and Harold organized the agenda of tactical and strategy issues to be discussed. The goal was to come up with a winning strategy to overcome the extreme bias we all faced.

I flew from San Francisco Airport to Wichita with a fellow trial lawyer handling many of these cases, Richard (Dick) Sangster. Dick was an accomplished northern California trial lawyer and a great person with whom to begin my brain storming weekend. As we flew to the middle of the country, Dick and I explored some meaningful strategy concepts that I subsequently put to use in the *Ahearn* trial.

Dick commented, "Sal, I think it would be a big mistake if the jury believes a favorable verdict would take the 'Pill' off the market."

"The belief that a plaintiff's verdict would take the 'Pill' off the market may explain the series of defense verdicts we've been seeing in these cases. My feeling is that our real theme should be *a woman's right to know* what risk she is taking when she puts that little pill in her mouth," I replied.

Dick confirmed, "That should definitely be our theme, let's share that with the better minds in Wichita when we get there."

Dick and I agreed this theme should be repeatedly emphasized, throughout a trial—that we are only arguing for a woman's right to know what are the risks to which she is being exposed when taking the "Pill," and the decision to take that risk or not is one between her and her physician—not that of the all-male Board of Directors of Johnson & Johnson.

We arrived at the hotel late in the evening, shared a drink with all the others who had arrived and then hit the sack. The next morning, we all met for breakfast, more than a dozen of us, before heading off to Gerry's office to begin the serious business of brainstorming. Fortunately, Gerry's office was close to the hotel so that we all spent minimum time at zero degrees F.

Gerry welcomed us all and thanked us for braving the trip to the cold of Wichita. Gerry Michaud was an exceptional trial lawyer with years of experience trying drug and medical malpractice cases throughout the Midwest. He excelled in cross-examination and had taken many of the depositions of key defense witnesses in "Pill" cases. He mastered the art of knowing when and how to go for the jugular of an adverse witness. This meeting would allow me the opportunity to see and review his depositions of key defense corporate personnel, some of which I could face in my trial. Some of Gerry's depositions would save me having to retake those same depositions in my case. It also would enhance my effectiveness over the defense, because they would not know I had those depositions available to impeach their witnesses at trial. In particular, I knew he had deposed Dr. Cronk, the medical director of Ortho, who was a key Defense witness. This would be a deposition I could heavily rely upon in preparing the *Ahearn* case for trial without the necessity to retake his deposition.

After Gerry's welcome, he stated, "We are here primarily to answer two questions. Why are we losing case after case before jurors? And what can we do to change that?"

Harold added his welcome to all of us and started the discussion on these key questions. During this meeting, I shared my views on how I thought we should approach the trial of these cases. This not only gave me the opportunity to test my strategy and tactics with some of the great minds in that room, but also learn from them as well. I shared the theme Richard Sangster and I discussed enroute to help us get around the fear in the minds of prospective jurors that a verdict for the plaintiff might end the availability of the "Pill." I suggested the real issue in the case was not that the "Pill" was bad and should be taken off the market. We knew that only *some* women were put at risk, even though there was no known way to identify who those women might be. Therefore, it was my strategy that the theme of oral contraceptive cases should be *"the right to know,"* i.e., that every woman had the right to know what the real risks of thrombosis were if they took the "Pill." They could then reasonably decide for themselves whether or not they wanted to take that risk. It should be a decision made between a woman and her doctor. In other words, in Michelle's case, it was her right to make such a decision with the advice of her doctor.

As I listened to the many comments from others about this theme, our discussions convinced me that Dick and I had stumbled upon the right theme that might reverse the losing streak. I knew the *Ahearn* case would be the test for this strategy since it would most likely be the next "Pill" case to proceed to trial within the United States.

Over the next two days we focused on the specific experts the pharmaceutical industry was using against us in our various cases. We brainstormed various approaches to use on cross-examination of these medical experts. I left Wichita, Kansas, with renewed confidence we had an excellent opportunity to turn the tide and produce a winner.

❧

As the trial date approached, the focus of many trial lawyers all over the country turned to the *Ahearn* case. All realized the nature of the injury alone, total blindness, would attract much newspaper publicity and shock the public into at least asking the question: Is the "Pill" really safe?

By this time Ortho's pressure of imposing constant discovery, depositions, motions, and such, unnecessarily increased our cost of pursuing litigation. Ortho knew it was a standard in the profession that personal injury cases are handled on a contingent fee basis. Thus, they increased the costs knowing that the burden would be entirely on the plaintiff lawyers, and if the case was lost, much of Ortho's costs could be recouped from the plaintiffs, themselves. This strategy often resulted in unfair low settlements or sometimes even abandonment of trial by a dismissal of the case.

Around this time my partner, Dick Caputo, was also feeling the effects of this increasing black cloud. Sensing that the risk of a loss was growing by leaps and bounds, he came to me one day expressing his concerns. He, too, was raising a young family and was quite averse to taking extraordinary risks. He explained he was losing sleep at night pondering the financial effect of a loss on the firm. I not only fully understood his quagmire and respected his serious concerns; I was open to any suggestions he had. Dick and I were not only partners, but very close friends. I started my first day of practice learning from him, ultimately becoming his partner. I was always aware that Dick was far more conservative toward risk taking than I. We ultimately reached an arrangement where Dick would no longer be exposed to a financial risk of loss in the case. The financial burden would be solely on me, however,

Dick continued to contribute invaluable insight to my handling of the case to its end.

Since Harold and I were doing all the work on the case, the only effect on me was to increase my personal financial risk, which I was more than willing to accept. After all, it was my urging that got us into the case, and I didn't feel that Dick should be forced to live with the emotional and financial circumstances that were being forced upon us.

To deal with this additional financial burden, with my wife, Laura's, consent and continual moral support, I refinanced my family home. Having been in practice for only ten years, I was therefore, more vulnerable to financial defeat than more established trial lawyers. In addition, we were raising our five children, ages three to thirteen years old, all in private schools. There was no doubt we were substantially increasing our personal financial risk by continuing the case. However, based upon all the evidence we had gathered by that time, concerning the catastrophic risks of the "Pill," in our minds, there was no turning back.

Knowing I was in the process of preparing to go to trial shortly, my pathologist friend, Dr. Paul Vincent gave me a call. Paul, Bill, and I had spent many hours discussing the medical aspects of this case.

"Sal, I'll be doing an autopsy tomorrow that I think would be very helpful to you if you scrubbed in. It will give you a better understanding of the critical anatomical structures involved in your *Ahearn* case. I should warn you, the decedent is a young woman which could be emotionally difficult for you to handle. Of necessity, I'll be dissecting the head and brain in my task of finding the cause of death. If you scrub in, you'll be able to visualize more clearly the structures important to you such as the pterygoid plexis, cavernous sinus area, as well as trace the two optic nerve pathways through the brain."

The timing could not have been more opportune. I knew I would be cross-examining some of the most knowledgeable medical experts in the country at this trial. This experience would give me the extra confidence in my own medical knowledge of those vital anatomical areas I would need to master in order to do an effective cross-examination.

"Thanks Paul, it sounds like a great opportunity. I can handle it, I'll be there."

Paul performed the autopsy in the usual procedure. As he dissected through human tissue, he would identify each anatomical structure and describe its condition into a recording microphone hanging over the cadaver body. I was not only able to observe each anatomical structure in its entirety but was also able to see how the structures were situated and interfaced with surrounding tissue. I observed how the venous and arterial systems interplayed with the cavernous sinus and the optic nerves as well as other vital structures. This was an incredibly timely learning experience.

Paul and my other pathology friend, Bill Siegel, were among the very few physicians who believed in the case. My wife's OB-GYN, Dr. Vince Nola, a good friend from my years at Bellarmine and Santa Clara University, also felt I was on target, and provided a lot of helpful, practical medical information to assist me, such as his inter-relationship, communications and experience with Ortho's detail men. He further related the lack of knowledge of thrombosis and the "Pill," among OB-GYNs in general, as experienced at medical conventions he had attended. The same was true of my own personal physician, Dr. Robert (Bob) Wilson. A respected board-certified Internist, Bob not only followed the case closely, but would ask me to share with him medical literature we had accumulated through our research to assist him in his practice— due the paucity of information on the "Pill" in the Physicians' Desk Reference provided by the pharmaceutical industry.

I was fortunate to have several good friends who were competent physicians in varied areas of expertise. Their continual moral support plus their contribution of medical knowledge kept me from being swallowed up by a black cloud of depression that surrounded this litigation. I had tremendous respect for their knowledge, competency, and integrity.

✍

Critical to any trial is the context of testimony by experts; they can make or break a case. With this awareness, I met with each of our potential expert witnesses to discuss their specific opinions and potential testimony, as well as further alert them what to expect during their cross-examination. I reviewed with them any medical studies and literature they would choose to rely upon at trial. To alleviate the risk of one of our experts contradicting another, I briefed them on who the other expert witnesses would be and the opinions they would be rendering. I brought them up to date as to the anticipated Defense experts and their expected testimony.

Harold and I made an appointment to meet with two of Michelle's most critical treating physicians, Dr. Sogg, her neuro-ophthalmologist, and Dr. Lippe, her neurosurgeon, to discuss their testifying on behalf of Michelle at trial.

Contrary to the usual treating doctor of a typical plaintiff in litigation, neither was very welcoming. They told us they did not believe the "Pill" caused Michelle's blindness. Rather, they believed her entire illness and ultimate blindness was all the result of an initial strep infection, probably starting in her throat.

In the course of the conversation, we learned something alarming to us both as plaintiff lawyers. A treating physician is ethically not expected to communicate with the opposite side of litigation concerning the medical issues of their patient, other than in the company of the patient's lawyer, or in a properly noticed deposition where the patient's lawyer is always present. Both of these treating doctors gave us the clear impression they had been communicating with the Defense, without our knowledge, nor their patient's consent. Further, they revealed to us they had agreed to testify against their own patient, Michelle, on behalf of the Defendant, Ortho. They each kept our meeting very brief and showed no interest in hearing our side of the evidence on the medical issues. It obviously appeared that their respective minds were clearly made up, and nothing we could say or do would change their views. Since jurors tend to accept the opinion of a treating physician over a retained expert, a "hired gun" in the vernacular, I knew we were in trouble from the start.

Harold, himself having once been a treating physician, was not as disturbed by this turn of events as I was.

I remarked to Harold, "Both Dr. Sogg and Dr. Lippe clearly harbor a strong dislike for me having brought this lawsuit. They clearly didn't appreciate my questioning their diagnosis of the cause, as a mere lawyer. They specifically didn't like my pointing out to them that nowhere in the hospital records did they even reference that Michelle had been on the "Pill" and resented my pointing out that they never even asked her during her entire hospitalization."

"I can understand that," Harold said.

"To me, they were obviously convinced, along with almost every other doctor in Santa Clara County who has been reading about our case in the local press, that I was just another greedy plaintiff lawyer creating another unmeritorious lawsuit."

Harold agreed.

Certain physicians were repeatedly quoted in the press condemning me for filing the lawsuit and pursuing such an unmeritorious case. The bias for the "Pill" was as powerful among physicians, particularly those who prescribed the "Pill," as it was among the public at large. This was the environment in which we would be trying this case. Harold agreed with my assessment. I noted to Harold, our clients were becoming particularly upset by the multitude of negative newspaper articles on the case.

∾

California law requires each side to timely identify each and every expert they intend to call to testify at trial, provide a copy of their curriculum vitae, and further identify each issue in the case that the particular expert will be called upon to present opinion testimony. Each party is thereby also given the opportunity to take the deposition of the others' experts. Obtaining their opinions, under oath, with their reasons is critical in most cases. One would think that such a tight procedure would eliminate any surprises at trial, it does not.

A major surprise arose in the trial testimony taken by way of deposition only a month and a half before the commencement of trial. We received a notice of a motion by Ortho seeking a court order to take an out-of-state deposition of Dr. Herbert Ley, a past FDA Commissioner, in Washington, D.C., as their trial witness. Since he was beyond subpoena range of a California court, the deposition could be taken as trial testimony to be read to the jury by Ortho at the actual trial. I became quite concerned when this occurred, assuming they would not do this if they didn't have this FDA commissioner in their hip pocket. Knowing that any opposition to this motion would fail, I stipulated to the order.

As I flew to Washington, D.C. to cross-examine him in the deposition, I frankly became scared of what might be yet to come. This deposition could severely damage our case if the commissioner took the position there was no evidence the "Pill" caused thrombosis in some women. After all, the FDA never *required* Ortho or the industry to provide such a warning in either the package insert or elsewhere. They, in fact, had the authority to do so. The big question was why didn't they? Harold was convinced that if placed under oath, Dr. Ley would admit causation. I was not so convinced. In fact, I was quite scared of what he might say, especially considering the prominence of an FDA Commissioner, from whom a jury would most likely accept any testimony he provided as true.

When I walked into the deposition room in a government building in Washington, D.C., I introduced myself to Dr. Ley before the deposition started and found him initially to be a warm and friendly gentleman. This did not lower my fear of what was to come.

Marion Pothoven, on behalf of Ortho, started the deposition by having Dr. Ley describe his educational and experience background. Dr. Ley's credentials were most impressive. A graduate of Harvard Medical School, postgraduate school with a Master's degree in Public Health (epidemiology), he served eleven years in the military performing medical research work. Subsequently, he became professor and chairman of the Department of Microbiology, Bacteriology, and Hygiene at George Washington School of Community Medicine. In 1963 he became an associate professor in Harvard School of Public Health until 1966 when he was hired by the FDA as Director of the Bureau of Medicine. From June 1968 until December 1969, Dr. Ley served as Commissioner of the FDA. He was a certified expert and specialist in preventive medicine and public health.

In his direct testimony, Marion had Dr. Ley summarize the history of warnings approved by the FDA. In 1964, the PDR (Physician's Desk Reference) widely used by prescribing physicians at the time, stated that "no serious side reactions to Ortho-Novum have been encountered." In 1965-1966, it stated that as to thrombosis ". . . there is no evidence to support a causal relationship . . ." In 1968, the warning was changed to "a statistical significant association" existing between the "Pill" and thrombosis. Basically, Marion had Dr. Ley confirm what the FDA was allowing the industry to say to doctors at that time to legitimize the industry's warnings.

As I began my cross-examination, his cooperative demeanor towards me changed the entire atmosphere in the room. It was almost like he wanted me to open up the door so the truth could come out.

"Doctor, can you provide more detail on the history of the FDA's involvement with the oral contraceptive industry?"

Dr. Ley explained, "In early 1968 the staff of the FDA and its OB-GYN advisory committee, in a conference with industry, recommended a change in the warnings contained in the package insert to reflect a *cause and effect* relationship between the "Pill" and thromboembolic disorders."

To my surprise, he then volunteered, "Ortho, in concert with other manufacturers, successfully opposed these changes by pressure brought upon certain FDA officials. The result was a compromised version having no reference to cause and effect, but rather the use of the epidemiological term a 'statistical significant association,' which is meaningless as to warning of a causal relationship to the typical prescribing physician."

Even this term did not appear in the package insert until July 1968, and had not reached Michelle's physician, Dr. Gossack, in time to alert him of anything.

During my cross-examination a second major shock surfaced in Dr. Ley's testimony.

"Dr. Ley, were the challenge and response cases reported to the FDA by industry?"

"No, the challenge and response cases were not reported to the FDA. I was advised of only one challenge and response case report prior to late 1969."

"Was there any significance to the challenge and responses cases to you and the FDA?"

"*Yes, these case reports constituted the final evidence to convince me of a cause and effect relationship in late 1969, after I had already succumbed to the industry position.* The combination of challenge and response cases, together with the retrospective studies, finally lead me to conclude that a cause and effect relationship did exist between the "Pill" and thrombosis."

Unfortunately, this was again too late to warn Michelle or her physician.

Dr. Ley further conceded the patient booklets that Ortho and other manufacturers handed out to women *"contained false and deliberately misleading statements"* and innuendoes about the safety of the "Pill" as disseminated to the public in 1965-1966 without FDA approval. He went on to testify that significant information concerning the safety of the "Pill" *was deleted from the package insert, the PDR, the doctor's file cards, and direct mail literature, in violation of federal regulations.*

I left Washington D.C. overjoyed. On my flight back, I thought about how we now had on record testimony from the FDA Commissioner, himself, that Ortho cheated and covered up the causal relationship. I found it incredible that Dr. Ley's testimony in that deposition was so powerful in support of Michelle's case. It was clear to me we should make him our own witness and we, not the Defense, should read it into evidence to the jury at trial.

I reflected on how our review of Ortho's records in Raritan, New Jersey, did not reveal any evidence of the 1968 conference of OB-GYNs with the FDA as described by Dr. Ley. We had learned from a deposition of Dr. Cronk, taken by Gerry Michaud, that Ortho deliberately destroyed all records and inter-office memoranda pertaining to this 1968 conference with the FDA when the "cause and effect" change in the language of the package insert was at issue. Yet, internal sales bulletins predating those years, but favorable to Ortho, were not destroyed.

I met with Michelle and Dennis at my office, again, to bring them up to date. Michelle was becoming scared now that they were facing an imminent trial date. The constant negative exposure by the press added to their fears. Michelle put it quite bluntly.

"I knew this was going to be difficult because you told us this many times. We're fighting a giant corporation and they're throwing out everything they have to beat you. I know this is one of the biggest cases coming up and I know this is going to be really hard. We have a David and Goliath story here. I know we have to do it, but don't know how it's going to come out."

Then, as had become Michelle's way when dealing with pressure in the case, she would joke or tease with me.

"Hey Sal, you know F. Lee Bailey, the big deal criminal attorney? Are you as good as F. Lee Bailey?"

I would jokingly reply, "Michelle, I am as good as he is, if not better!"

"Okay, you're my F. Lee Bailey."

CHAPTER 6
THE JURY

There does not exist a single institution on the planet, created by man or woman wherein the truth has a more probable chance of surfacing than in a court of law within the United States of America. Although not perfect, the Rule of Law, rather than the rule of man, still prevails. If we should ever lose that, truth will forever evade us.

Throughout the pretrial process, a variety of different judges decide motions and resolve conflicting issues. Now that our trial date was upon us, we were faced with a major determination— who will be the judge that tries this case? The lawyers involved do not get to select the judge. The assignment of a judge to a particular case is made by the presiding judge of the county.

On the morning of October 28, 1974, Harold and I, along with Marion Pothoven and the Defense team, appeared before the Presiding Judge to be assigned a trial judge for the *Ahearn* case. The case of *Ahearn vs. Johnson & Johnson, et al.* was then duly assigned to Judge Bruce F. Allen, an experienced trial judge who had been on the Superior Court of Santa Clara County for several years.

The role of a trial judge in a jury trial is even more important than the jury itself. The trial judge's duty is not merely to ensure the orderly presentation of evidence and conformance with the law of evidence. The judge has a further duty to instruct the jury on the law that applies to the case. Although each side submits to the court their version of jury instructions they believe should be given to the jury, disagreements between the parties occur, and are ultimately resolved by the trial judge. The judge, in effect, makes the ultimate decision as to what will be the law applied to this case. The jury decides what are the true facts.

Having been told by the Presiding Judge that Judge Allen would be our trial judge, each side now had their only opportunity to object to the assignment by filing an affidavit asserting that Judge Allen could not be fair and unbiased in this case. My only previous experience with Judge Allen was various motions and matters pertaining to other cases including one other jury trial. I found him to be fair and unbiased in the past and therefore had no objection to him. The Defense did not object as well, so Judge Allen became our trial judge. Once Judge Allen began any proceedings over the case, that right to challenge is thereafter waived. Despite my comfortable feelings, some local trial lawyers referred to him as *unpredictable* and by a few, a *maverick*.

Unlike with a jury, a trial lawyer does not have the opportunity to voir dire the judge to seek out any bias or prejudice to the particular issues in that specific case. I could not ask Judge Allen if he had any set opinion on the birth control pill and its risks. Judges, as with all of us human beings, have biases and prejudices.

The concern is: do any of these biases or prejudices have any relevance to this particular case? The law provides the judge must recuse himself from the case if he recognizes he may have a bias or prejudice to any party or issue in the case. Obviously Judge Allen did not.

Assigned to Judge Allen, Harold, Michelle, Dennis and I made our way to his courtroom on the next floor. Upon arrival, his clerk immediately informed us that the Judge wanted to see counsel for both sides in his chambers. This was normal procedure. The court uses such opportunity to learn from the lawyers what the case involves and some of the key issues. This also gives the judge the opportunity to determine if there might be any conflict of interest or bias in his handling the case, and if so to recuse himself at that point.

I told Michele and Dennis to wait in the courtroom while we all met with the judge. I explained judges typically just want to discuss the anticipated length of trial and the nature of the case with the attorneys alone.

Judge Allen initially greeted us cordially as was his customary style. He asked what the case was about and what were the essential issues.

"Your Honor, our contention is that our client, Michelle Ahearn, was blinded from blood clotting caused by Ortho-Novum, manufactured by Ortho, a subsidiary of Johnson & Johnson."

Marion then contributed from the Defense viewpoint, "Ortho's contention is that it was a strep infection and not their product that caused her blindness, or it was just an idiopathic, spontaneous clotting episode that can occur in any human being."

Judge Allen's immediately responded.

"I realize that if you made a study you will find a certain amount of people who are poisoned by table salt . . . certain number of people can be poisoned by sodium glutamate . . . juries are easily swayed in this type of case."

Harold and I stood there, shocked at what we heard. We became very uncomfortable realizing we were now stuck with Judge Allen for the entire trial. Our opportunity to challenge him had passed. Our only hope was that he would be swayed by what we believed was overwhelming evidence in support of our contention, that the "Pill" caused Michelle's blindness.

We walked out of the judge's chambers toward the courtroom and Michelle asked me what happened. I told her what the Judge had said, but added, "He hasn't heard any of the evidence, so he has no idea how strong and persuasive it is," not wanting to unsettle them. Harold and I, however, realized we had a potential problem with this judge in addition to a complex difficult trial.

∽

We returned to the courtroom and took our respective seats at counsel table. Judge Allen ordered the bailiff to bring up the first group of potential jurors from the jury assembly room on the first floor of the courthouse and turned to us saying, "Are you ready to start jury selection?"

"Yes, your Honor," Marion and I responded.

The role of a juror in an American trial is to be the judge as to what the true facts are in the case, and then apply the law to those facts, as instructed to them by the judge. Such becomes their "verdict." The word *verdict* is derived from the ancient Latin and original French which means "to say the truth" or "to speak the truth." The word succinctly sums up the purpose of the sworn duty of a jury in an American trial, whether civil or criminal, i.e., to find the truth and say the truth through their verdict, in the verdict form they sign and submit to the court at the end of a trial. For this reason, a verdict carries substantial respect in the law, and cannot be overturned for minor or irrelevant reasons.

As the sole judge of the facts, the ideal juror should be a person who carries absolutely no bias or prejudice with regard to the issues in the case. The juror must be intelligent enough and mentally capable to understand the facts and the pertinent issues. Last, but not least in my view, such juror must have the courage and fortitude to vote from their conscience in judging those facts, and not be swayed by any prior prejudice, understanding, or popular belief.

In the *Ahearn* case, it was my goal to select the most educated jurors available to me. I was less concerned whether they were conservative or liberal, Republicans, Independents, or Democrats, as long as they would be competent enough to see through the Big Pharma propaganda I anticipated.

Court proceedings began. The bailiff escorted fifty prospective jurors into Judge Allen's courtroom. The Judge welcomed the prospective jurors and advised them that this was a civil case estimated to possibly last as long as two months which would take it into the Christmas holiday season. Judge Allen then began the process of questioning those individual prospective jurors who requested to be excused due to hardship or any other reason that made it difficult or impossible to serve in such a long case. This process eliminated so many that another group of fifty prospective jurors had to be called up from the jury assembly room.

After reaching a sufficient number of those not excused for hardship, Judge Allen then gave each juror a written questionnaire form of several pages pertaining to personal and very sensitive matters regarding each prospective juror's background, education, employment history, life experiences, and more that might be relevant to the issues in this case. This questionnaire was prepared by each side reaching an agreement on every question together with the Judge's approval. Included were questions as to whether, if female, the juror was on or had ever been on oral contraceptives or used any other type of birth control, and, if male, as to their respective spouse. It also inquired as to any specific knowledge such juror possessed pertaining to oral contraceptives, specifically as to any side effects or warnings that may have come to their attention. These questionnaires were ordered to be held strictly confidential but made a part of the official court record.

Every prospective juror having completed the confidential questionnaire, the Clerk of the Court then randomly pulled from a box the name of the first twelve jurors to be seated in the jury box, together with three alternates. The oral voir dire process (questioning) by the lawyers for each side then began in open court on the usual voir dire issues, such as more detail on educational background not revealed in the questionnaire, or attitude toward lawsuits such as this, awarding damages for pain and suffering, and such. Thereafter each prospective juror was further questioned by the lawyers in Judge Allen's chambers, out of the hearing of the other jurors and the public attending the trial, on the more sensitive and private issues pertaining to oral contraceptive or other birth control use, experience, and side effects.

We reached the end of the day and the Court recessed. As we walked out of the courtroom, I asked Michelle how she felt about the jurors selected so far, and if her woman's intuition made her feel uncomfortable about any juror sitting in the jury box.

"I've never been in a courtroom before, not even for a traffic ticket. This is all new and scary and tremendously intimidating to me. I can't believe how tedious this is, how much effort you and the Defense put into selecting the jury—with all the questions, trying to decide their demeanor and answers, whether you would accept them or not, and how important it is. I was never aware of how important this is until now. You told me to tell you if any juror didn't sound right to me. When you said that, I thought to myself, 'What do I know?' You know what you are doing. What am I going to do, tell you I don't like this person's voice and mess things up?"

We returned the next day and continued with extensive questioning until all the prospective jurors had been thoroughly vetted for any bias or prejudice that might affect their judging this case.

The Court then asked if either side had any challenge for *cause* on any juror. A typical challenge for cause exists if the prospective juror admits they cannot be fair to both sides in this particular case due to some personal bias or prejudice relating to the issues or parties. The judge will then excuse such juror for cause. This occurred when two jurors acknowledged, after extensive questioning, that they could not be fair and impartial.

The Court then invited me, as Plaintiffs' counsel, to exercise any peremptory challenge I might have on any of the jurors sitting in the jury box at that moment. Each side was given eight peremptory challenges, which meant that each side can remove from the jury up to eight prospective jurors, without stating any cause or reason to the Judge.

I responded, "Plaintiffs would thank and excuse Juror No. 5, your Honor."

Having excused that juror, the Court then invited the Defense to exercise its peremptory challenge, and back and forth until each of us had exercised all eight peremptory challenges that we were allowed. Ultimately, after two days of questioning, a jury of twelve plus three alternate jurors were selected and sworn in as jurors.

In a civil case, under California law, for the jury to reach a verdict, at least nine out of twelve must agree. If all the alternates are used and a further juror becomes ill, it could lead to a mistrial. The case would then have to be retried from the beginning before a new jury. This potential made three alternate jurors a necessity in the *Ahearn* case.

The educational level of the ultimate jury panel was astonishing. The ultimate juror chosen to be the foreperson of the jury, whose job was to maintain an orderly and fair process during the deliberations in the jury room, was the most educated of all. She studied medicine, was trained in epidemiology (medical statistics), attained a degree in psychology, worked as a psychological examiner, and attained a master's degree in child development, which she taught as a member of a college faculty. She was a prolific reader of professional and scientific journals and reports, many obtained through her husband, a professor of chemistry at a local university, and her son, a medical student. She had read many articles on the "Pill" as well. The Defense had thoroughly examined her on all of this during voir dire and accepted her as a fair juror in this case and so did we.

Another female juror had two years of college at the University of California, Berkeley in English and child development, and her husband owned and managed a major auto dealership which was a large corporation. In voir dire examination she described how her husband was often sued. She also admitted to having been on the "Pill" at one time and experiencing minor side effects.

Five other jurors were college graduates, and five others had some college education. The remaining two completed high school. Two had special training in medicine, one of which was a registered nurse, the other a pre-med student and a psychologist. Their combined education and experience exceeded that of most jurors, attorneys, and even judges in the scientific areas that related to the factual issues involved in this case.

After the jury was sworn, Judge Allen did something very unusual that shocked us, as well as the Defense. He told the jury that each juror would be allowed to individually question, orally in open court, each witness that testifies, but only after each attorney and the Court had finished their respective questioning.

In 56 years of trying cases, this is the only trial I have experienced where oral open court questioning of witnesses by jurors has ever been allowed. The usual procedure has always been to allow the juror to submit written questions to the judge who, after review with the attorneys on each side, would decide whether to answer that question in open court, or allow the witness to answer it.

This unusual procedure concerned not only Harold and I, but Marion Pothoven and his assisting lawyers as well. If some juror should unknowingly ask a question not allowed under the rules of evidence, or in itself demonstrated a bias or prejudice to either side, would we then be faced with a mistrial and have to start the trial all over again? Both Marion and I looked at each other wondering how could we stop this? Of course, neither of us dared make an objection in front of the jury, for fear the jury would then think we were trying to hide something by preventing them from asking questions.

Judge Allen then gave a customary brief description of the case to the jury as previously agreed to by the attorneys. He informed the jury that the Plaintiff, Michelle Ahearn, contends she was injured consuming Ortho-Novum manufactured and sold by the Defendants, Ortho-Pharmaceutical Corporation, Johnson & Johnson, and Lucky Stores Inc., and further that her husband, Dennis Ahearn, claimed a loss of consortium therefrom. He informed them that the Defendants denied all such claims.

Thereafter, the judge allowed us to distribute to each juror a glossary of medical terms[3] that would be commonly referred to by expert witnesses during testimony to assist them in following the complicated medical issues in the case. The jurors utilized this glossary extensively throughout the case and found it invaluable in assisting them in following the expert testimony.

The judge then gave them some initial instructions on their duties as jurors.

"Now, the jury is the sole judge of the facts. This means that it is up to you as jurors to decide what happened. And this involves deciding what witnesses you believe or do not believe. You might decide you don't believe any of it or some of it or all of it, because

---

3   Appendix A contains the Medical Glossary the jury was given.

that is the jury's job . . . it will be up to you to decide what opinions you wish to accept or reject because again that is a jury's job."

This important instruction would play a major role in the outcome of the case.

The judge explained that the plaintiff would give an opening statement describing the facts in the case from their viewpoint followed by an opening statement by the defendant. Next, the plaintiff would present its witnesses and evidence first because the plaintiff has the burden of proof. The "burden of proof" in a civil action requires that the plaintiff prove its case by a "preponderance of evidence," i.e., by a greater weight of the evidence, that the plaintiff's contentions are "more probable than not." Then the defense would present its witnesses and counter evidence followed by each side presenting final arguments.

Judge Allen encouraged the jury's willingness to participate by telling them that this trial would be an opportunity for them "not only to serve on a jury, but to get a good medical education in certain aspects of medicine or drugs."

He then recessed for the day and ordered the jury back to Court the next morning to begin the actual trial.

CHAPTER 7
TRIAL BEGINS

The primary and most difficult task of a trial lawyer in the course of trial is to reduce the complex technical factual information to a level that is understandable to a lay jury, through the process of questioning expert and lay witnesses. In short, the trial lawyer is a teacher in the courtroom and the lay jurors are the students. The subject matter, no matter how complicated, must be taught through the process of direct and cross-examination of the witnesses using understandable demonstrative evidence. The complex science and medical issues in the *Ahearn* case presented a major challenge to this difficult task.

With a jury finally selected, Harold and I headed to Court on October 30, 1974 to begin the actual trial. We met up with Michelle and Dennis as we entered the courthouse. I explained to Michelle and Dennis we were quite pleased with jury composition, especially being able to succeed with nine women on a case with such crucial women's issues, as well as the overall educational level.

Together we walked down the hallway of the second floor of the courthouse. As we approached Judge Allen's courtroom, we walked past the waiting jurors. Entering, I noticed a large number of people present in the gallery to observe the trial, including a reporter for the *San Jose Mercury*, several lawyers whom I knew, my wife Laura, and my father, Sam.

The austerity of the courtroom with its light wood paneling, large gallery, wood bar railing separating the gallery with spectators from the official court personnel, lawyers, jurors, and potential witnesses, created an imposing atmosphere.

Harold and I wheeled in our carts, stacked three to four banker boxes high containing documents critical to the trial. I directed Michelle and Dennis to sit in the first two seats on the jury side of the gallery, just behind the bar railing. I explained these would be their permanent seats throughout the trial. That location provided the simplest communication access among us.

We then took our seats at the counsel table closest to the jury box as is traditional for plaintiffs' counsel in a civil case and I began organizing my notes for opening statement. On the opposite counsel table, Marion and his two associate lawyers did the same. Marion and I each had our paralegals seated in the first row of the gallery, likewise, for easy communication access.

After we situated ourselves, Judge Allen's bailiff then went out into the hallway and summoned the jurors to the courtroom. There was a quiet solemnity as each juror entered the jury box and took their assigned seat. At this point, as I glanced back at the gallery, I noticed my wife, Laura, rise and leave the courtroom. I thought it strange in that we were about to begin with opening statements.

"All rise. The Honorable Bruce S. Allen, presiding," the Bailiff announced as Judge Allen briskly entered the courtroom from his chambers in his black robes and took his seat at the bench.

Judge Allen turned to the jury. "Good morning, ladies and gentlemen."

He turned back toward the counsel table and we all exchanged morning greetings. He then requested counsel to approach the bench for a discussion out of the hearing of the jury. He advised us Juror #1 had called in sick and we would have to replace that juror with Alternate #1. Marion and I agreed to that obvious necessity and returned to counsel table. The judge then explained the situation to the jury. He indicated this demonstrated the importance of having alternate jurors available. However, I became concerned that we had lost a juror so early in the trial.

Judge Allen then addressed the jury.

"We will now hear an opening statement from Plaintiffs' counsel and possibly one from the defense. The opening statement is not evidence, but it is helpful in introducing the facts of the case to you. Any statement by the attorneys is not evidence and should not be taken as such. The only evidence is what comes from sworn witnesses on the witness stand and documents admitted into evidence."

Judge Allen addressed Harold and I, "Counsel, you can proceed with your opening statement."

In opening statements, we were prohibited from arguing the case, we could only present the facts we believed we could prove. The primary purpose was to paint for the jury the big picture of the case, so that when they heard testimony they would know how and where it related to the factual issues involved.

I began my opening statement on behalf of Michelle and Dennis:

"Ladies and gentlemen, I want to thank each of you for bearing with us through an extensive voir dire examination that involved your very personal and private information. However, at the end of the trial when you enter the jury room and start your deliberations, you will then realize and appreciate the necessity of such questioning. This is my opportunity to discuss with you the factual background of this case and the factual evidence we believe the testimony from our experts will show in support of our contention that the "Pill" caused Michelle's blindness, and that the Defendants violated their duty to warn. We do not contend that the "Pill" was the only cause, but rather that it was *a cause* among others, *a substantial factor* in causing Michelle's blindness. We are not saying the "Pill" is a defective drug and, therefore, should not have been put on the market for human consumption. What we are saying in this case, is that a woman has a right to know as well as her physician, what are the real risks of taking this drug?"

I emphasized to the jury that the facts would show that Michelle and her doctor were intentionally deprived of knowing the risk of thrombosis that would have allowed her, together with her doctor, to make their own decision as to whether she should take that risk. I narrowed the issues down to the following, which I had prepared on a large white sheet of paper on an easel for the jury to see:

1. Does the "Pill" cause abnormal clotting of blood—thrombosis and thrombophlebitis in some women?

2. If so, was *thrombosis* a substantial factor in causing Michelle's blindness?

3. If so, was *the "Pill"* a substantial factor in causing the thrombosis in Michelle?

4. If so, were the warnings by the Defendants adequate?

5. If not, did Ortho know the warnings were inadequate?

I briefly discussed what the evidence would be regarding Ortho's pre-marketing and post-marketing testing. I specifically pointed out to the jury the selection of a clinical director located in El Paso, Texas, Dr. Goldzeirher, who was heavily relied upon by Ortho in justifying their claim that their studies proved no causal link between the "Pill" and thrombosis.

"I presume the Defense will bring Dr. Goldzeirher to testify about his studies." I said this though I knew he was not on the Defense witness list.

I concluded with Michelle's story that would be placed in evidence, ending my opening statement with a vivid description of Michelle's life as a blind wife and mother with three children.

⌒♊⌒

The Defense was then allowed to present their opening statement. Marion told the jury what the evidence would be on the history of the "Pill," the magic of *ethinyl estradiol* in preventing unwanted pregnancies, the worldwide acceptance and use of the "Pill" as a simple, safe contraceptive. He contended there was no evidence that proved, by a greater probability, that the "Pill" was the cause of Michelle's blindness, and further that their extremely qualified experts would present scientific evidence that the "Pill" had not been proven to cause thrombosis in anyone. Marion emphasized that millions of women had been on the "Pill" all over the world and only a handful of anecdotal thrombosis cases of women on the "Pill" had been reported in the medical literature. Further, he contended the factual evidence from their extensive pre-marketing and post-marketing studies showed no evidence of causation between the "Pill" and thrombosis in any human being. He especially touted the extensive pre-marketing prospective studies performed in Texas by Dr. Goldzeirher in his major clinic having been specifically retained by Ortho.

Marion contended their medical experts would prove that Michelle's blindness was caused solely from a strep infection in the throat. Specifically, he emphasized an Ear, Nose and Throat (ENT) specialist from the Midwest, Dr. McCabe, who would provide this evidence. Dr. McCabe's expertise, Marion boasted, was on the anatomy of the human skull. "He has performed over a thousand surgeries on the human skull, itself."

Opening statements having taken a good part of the day, Judge Allen allowed us to recess until the following morning to commence with the presentation of live witnesses.

As we left the courtroom, I mentioned to Michelle and Dennis, "You now have heard the big picture of the battleground of your case. You can see the Defense is not going to roll over, however, wait until you hear our first witness."

They both expressed their gratitude for our extensive preparation and what they felt was a good opening statement, but were still perplexed being completely unfamiliar with the complexities of a trial.

Harold and I returned to my office to prepare for the next day. Our minds shifted to a crucial concern in every trial—the order of witnesses. There is a well-recognized psychological principle that people generally remember best what they hear at the beginning and at the end of a presentation. This concept of "primacy and recency" plays a major role in every trial, particularly in the order that witnesses are presented. Even though faced with the practical difficulty involving witnesses' availability, particularly with medical expert witnesses, we had struggled to ensure we would begin the trial with testimony that displayed some of the most powerful evidence in the case.

To this end, I subpoenaed in advance, Dr. Harris, to appear in Court at 9:00 a.m. the next morning. As to the remaining witnesses, now that we knew the certainty of the beginning of trial testimony, Harold and I got on the phone with them to reschedule their testimony.

I rushed home wondering why Laura had left the courtroom that morning as I began the opening statement. When I arrived home, she told me what happened.

"As I watched the jury walk in to take their seats in the jury box, I recognized a high school classmate of mine as one of your jurors. I realized that if she connected me to be your wife, that would create a mistrial. So I thought it best I leave the courtroom before she spotted me."

"Wow, am I grateful you had the wisdom to do that. That definitely could have led to a mistrial resulting in a loss of this jury I really like. I'd hate to have to start over again picking a new jury. You saved the day."

After dinner, I went back to work shifting my mind to the presentation of our witnesses.

As the judge mentioned, the first witnesses to testify are presented by the plaintiff because the plaintiff has the burden of proof under the law. The defense does not have to prove anything, but merely attack and weaken the plaintiff's case to the level where it no longer meets the burden of greater probability.

DONALD G. HARRIS, M.D.

I then began my preparation of the detail notes for direct examination of Dr. Harris.

I chose to begin with what I thought was one of the strongest pieces of evidence in the case—testimony that would surprise the Defense and overwhelm the jury with its persuasive power as well. I anticipated that the Defense would not know, or recall, Dr. Harris or his past written communications with Ortho.

The next morning on my way to the courthouse I had the usual qualms: will Dr. Harris show up even though he was subpoenaed? That's always a concern in a major trial, particularly with medical experts and their susceptibility to emergency situations. As I arrived, I met up with Harold, Michelle and Dennis as we entered the courthouse and made our way to Judge Allen's courtroom.

I was relieved to see Dr. Harris present.

"Good morning, Dr. Harris," I greeted him. "I appreciate you being here and will keep your testimony as short as possible You will be the first witness on the stand."

We settled in at counsel table waiting as Judge Allen entered. He took his position at the bench and extended his greetings to the jury and counsel, then addressed me.

"Counsel, are you ready to present your first witness?"

"Yes, your Honor, Plaintiffs would like to call Dr. Harris to the stand."

Marion popped up out of his chair, "Objection, your Honor. Dr. Harris is a medical doctor and was never identified as an expert witness."

As I had hoped, Marion was caught by surprise. He had no apparent knowledge of who Dr. Harris was, or why I was calling him as a witness. He assumed he would be testifying as an expert with opinions on the "Pill."

"We had no opportunity to take his deposition as to his expert opinions in his case and, therefore, he should not be allowed to testify under the law."

Addressing Judge Allen, I responded to Marion's objection.

"Your Honor, he is not being called as an expert witness to render any expert opinion testimony but will testify solely as a factual witness to authenticate certain documents for admission into evidence, as well as to respond to certain factual questions. Further, your Honor, he is not appearing voluntarily, he is here under subpoena."

"Objection overruled," said Judge Allen. "Dr. Harris will be allowed to testify as a factual witness only."

"Good morning, Dr. Harris. Would you describe your medical background for the jury?"

"I am a California licensed physician, board-certified in internal medicine, and in private practice in Mt. View, California, since 1959. I have been in private practice for more than fifteen years."

"Doctor, let me hand you a letter and ask you if you can identify it?"

"Yes, it's a letter I wrote to Dr. Cronk, the medical director for Ortho Pharmaceutical Corp. in 1967."

"Would you please read it to the jury?"

In the letter he described his patient who was the mother of six children, with no prior history of thrombosis or phlebitis, for whom he had prescribed Ortho-Novum, Ortho's "Pill." Within a very short time she developed thrombophlebitis in her leg. He took her off the "Pill," treated her, and she recovered uneventfully. He asked Dr. Cronk if there could be any relationship between Ortho-Novum and her developing thrombophlebitis.

"Doctor, let me show you a second letter and ask if you can identify it?"

"Yes, this is the response from Dr. Cronk to my letter."

"Please read that letter to the jury."

He read how Dr. Cronk denied any evidence existed demonstrating any causal relationship whatsoever between Ortho-Novum and thrombophlebitis. Dr. Cronk went on to describe the extensive pre-marketing and post-marketing testing Ortho had done, contending such studies proved no causal relationship *whatsoever* between their product and blood clotting of any type.

He also emphasized its safe use in millions of women over several years.

"Doctor, let me show you a third letter to identify. Is this your response to Dr. Cronk?"

"Yes, this is my second letter to Dr. Cronk."

"Please read that letter to the jury, as well."

The letter reflected that Dr. Harris had relied on Dr. Cronk's previous denial of a causal relationship between the "Pill" and blood clotting and, therefore, Dr. Harris had put his patient back on the "Pill" for a *second time*. She shortly thereafter developed thrombophlebitis again. He explained that he immediately took her off the "Pill" treated her, and she again recovered without any complications. In the letter he repeated his request for any information whatsoever that Ortho might possess concerning *any* possible relationship between the "Pill" and blood clotting disorders.

"Doctor, did you receive a response from your second letter to Dr. Cronk?"

"Yes."

"Is this Dr. Cronk's response to that second letter?"

He carefully reviewed the letter and responded, "Yes."

"Please read that letter to the jury."

He read that Dr. Cronk again stated that Ortho-Novum had been thoroughly tested, approved bythe FDA, and had been in use for several years in over a million women, and absolutely no evidence of a causal relationship ever surfaced. In the letter Dr. Cronk challenged Dr. Harris that he must not have obtained a thorough enough history from his patient. If he had, he would probably have found that his patient had a past history of spontaneous thrombophlebitis before ever taking Ortho-Novum.

"Dr. Harris, did you respond to Dr. Cronk's last letter?"

"Yes."

"Is this your response?"

He quickly glanced over the letters and responded, "Yes."

"Please read it to the jury."

In his *third letter* to Dr. Cronk, Dr. Harris described how Dr. Cronk's recent response was so convincing to the effect that no causal relationship existed, he placed his patient on the "Pill" for a *third* time. This time, his patient developed a blood clot that traveled to her lungs threatening her life. Emergency hospitalization saved her life and she eventually fully recovered. He again took her off the "Pill," permanently, and no further blood clotting disorders occurred. In this response, Dr. Harris attacked Dr. Cronk's assertion in his previous letter that he, Dr. Harris, did not know the medical history of his patient as being susceptible to thrombophlebitis. "The patient," he pointed out in the letter, "is my wife!"

Not surprisingly, the Defense waived cross-examination of Dr. Harris.

"Doctor Harris, thank you very much for responding to the subpoena and providing your factual testimony to this jury. Your Honor, may this witness be excused?"

Judge Allen excused Dr. Harris and I relaxed; the strategy worked. The jury heard firsthand from this physician who experienced this *triple challenge and response* which no physician or scientist involved with the "Pill" had yet experienced to that date. This November 1974 moment in a courtroom in San Jose, California, was the first public disclosure of this particular powerful scientific evidence of causation between the "Pill" and thrombosis.

HERBERT LEY, M.D.

Judge Allen turned toward me, "Counsel, please call your next witness."

"Your Honor, the next witness, Dr. Ley, will be presented by deposition testimony in that he is unavailable to testify in person as he resides in Washington, D.C. The Defendant Ortho requested that this deposition be taken as trial testimony in their case, however, we adopt his testimony and want to submit it in our case in chief. May I have my associate counsel, Harold Williams, take the stand to read Dr. Ley's responses as I read the questions?"

Judge Allen responded, "You may do so."

Harold walked over to the witness stand and took the seat with a copy of Dr. Ley's deposition in hand. I then read each question and Harold read the reply.

As with all expert witnesses, it is extremely important and significant to lay out their educational background and qualifications to provide credibility and support to their opinions. It is the jury's role to judge whether these qualifications justify the expert's opinions.

After providing Dr. Ley's extensive qualifications,[4] the jury heard this witness, who was the commissioner of the FDA at the time Michelle went blind, testify that he became convinced there was truly a cause and effect relationship between the "Pill" and thrombosis. They further heard his sworn testimony of the

---

4   For his qualifications and opinions see Dr. Ley's deposition discussed in Chapter 5.

influence Ortho and the industry brought upon FDA officials to prevent such a warning from getting to the medical world.

They heard his testimony that the combination of *challenge and response* cases together with the retrospective studies performed to date led him to the conclusion that a *cause and effect* relationship existed between the "Pill" and thrombosis. Retrospective studies are those performed by looking rearwards at the medical records of those in the study, as contrasted with prospective studies which look forward and follow the population being studied to determine any adverse reactions. Of significance is that Dr. Ley reached his scientific opinion on the "Pill" before knowing about Dr. Harris's triple challenge and response case.

Unfortunately, this evidence came to his attention too late to save Michelle. Prior to learning of the challenge and response cases (known to industry, but not reported to the FDA), his testimony explained how Dr. Ley was subjected to the pressure of industry to allow a watered down warning that the relationship was only a "statistical significant association," with no reference whatsoever to "cause and effect." Dr. Ley had noted that Dr. Harris' particular triple challenge and response case *had not been reported to the FDA as it should have been.*

Upon the completion of reading Dr. Ley's deposition testimony, Judge Allen recessed for lunch.

ROBERT MCCLEERY, M.D.

Harold and I met Dr. McCleery who had arrived in the courtroom and the three of us went to lunch to discuss his testimony. We felt anxious to get before the jury our next FDA witness. His live testimony would corroborate Dr. Ley's deposition testimony. Live testimony always carries more persuasive weight with a jury than merely reading the transcript of a deposition, which can put a jury to sleep no matter how powerful the testimony may be.

Harold met Dr. McCleery a few years earlier and had worked with him in preparing him to testify in earlier trials. I had not personally met him until this case and found him to be exceptionally qualified with powerful factual and scientific evidence of the risks of the "Pill." He also possessed a wealth of factual evidence of the industry's attempt to *cover-up* the thrombosis risk. His only weakness as a witness was his dry, monotone, voice and lack of any emotional expression. His boring voice could put a jury to sleep easily. I would have to get quite creative to keep his voice alive as well as his personality, but the substance of what he had to say was dynamite.

As we returned to the courtroom after lunch, I felt Dr. McCleery was well prepared to testify. Judge Allen took the bench and looking at me, said, "Counsel, call your next witness."

"Your Honor, the Plaintiffs call Dr. Robert McCleery to the stand as our next witness." As he walked to the stand, the jury was visibly relieved to see a live witness rather than the reading of another deposition.

"Dr. McCleery, please describe for the jury your medical education and background."

He described his specialty as a vascular surgeon with many years' experience as a practicing physician, medical school professor, and a writer of medical prescription drug advertising. He explained his six years with the FDA, monitoring information disseminated by manufacturers on the "Pill" as his immediate and primary responsibility, including the advertising books and pamphlets disseminated by Johnson & Johnson and Ortho Pharmaceutical Corporation.

"Doctor, while you were at the FDA, did the staff of medical doctors ever reach an opinion that there was a cause and effect relationship between the "Pill" and thrombosis?"

He responded in his monotone voice, "The entire FDA staff of medical doctors and their OB-GYN Advisory Committee had reached an opinion in early 1968 of a *cause and effect* relationship between the 'Pill' and thrombosis."

This was more than one year before Michelle suffered her life-threatening thrombosis and blindness.

"Doctor, were there any attempts to modify the warning to cause and effect language?"

"Attempts to modify the warnings to doctors and the public failed due to the manufacturer's *strong, prolonged and vigorous* opposition."

"Doctor, can you give us any approximate time period as to when this opposition occurred?"

"During meetings between the FDA and industry, on March 29 and May 8, 1968."

"Doctor, did Ortho Pharmaceutical participate at either of those meetings?"

"Yes, they were present and heavily participated at both meetings."

Dr. McCleery then went on to explain that he personally never changed his opinion that a *cause and effect* relationship did exist.

"How did the 'statistical significance association' language come about?"

"It was compromised language imposed by the pressure of industry."

"Do you have an opinion as to whether 'statistical significance association' is an adequate warning to physicians?"

"In my opinion, with my expertise in prescription drug advertising, I consider 'statistical significance association' as inadequate and completely meaningless to physicians as well as most women on the 'Pill.'"

He testified how patient booklets containing false and deliberate misleading statements and innuendoes as to the safety of the "Pill" were disseminated to the public in 1965-1969 *without FDA clearance and approval, as required by law.* Significant information concerning the safety of the "Pill" was deleted from the package insert (contained within the drug package), the PDR (Physicians' Desk Reference, which was a major source of reference on a prescription drug for physicians) and the doctor's file card personally delivered to the doctor by the pharmaceutical representative. He testified that *all were in violation of federal regulations.*

"Doctor, are you familiar with the extensive published studies performed in Great Britain mentioned in Ortho's package insert and the PDR?"

"Yes, I'm quite familiar with those studies which clearly provided evidence of a causal relationship between the 'Pill' and thrombosis."

"Doctor, were those studies mentioned by Ortho in their package insert?"

"Yes, they mention the studies but then claim that because they were done in Great Britain, the conclusions are *not* applicable to American women."

"Do you have an opinion as to whether or not that's a true statement?"

"Ortho never gave a rational explanation as to why it is not equally applicable to American women nor does any exist. It is a completely false and deliberate misleading statement."

On cross-examination, Marion couldn't make any points with Dr. McCleery, nor touch the veracity of any of his testimony. He was as experienced and competent as a witness as he was in his work with the FDA. The effect of cross-examination only highlighted the integrity and honesty of this expert FDA employee, and his disgust with the system's inability to prevent such misinformation reaching physicians and the public. He was truly unimpeachable.

Dr. McCleery ended the day's testimony. Judge Allen then dismissed the jury but requested counsel on both sides to remain in the courtroom to discuss some further matters.

In every trial, there are always issues to be discussed with the judge outside the presence of the jury as well as questions by the judge, such as the number of witnesses left to anticipate on both sides. Further, this provided the opportunity for us to convey to Marion and the Defense the anticipated witnesses for the next couple of days pursuant to a previous Court Order.

Following these discussions, we recessed until the next morning. Harold and I gathered up our materials and I asked Dennis and Michelle if they would like to meet us for dinner that evening to discuss the day's testimony. Harold and I then took Dr.

McCleery back to his hotel where he arranged his flight to return to Washington, D.C.

That evening Harold and I met with Michelle and Dennis for dinner at a favorite restaurant to discuss the progress of trial. This would become a somewhat frequent custom during the trial as a pleasant way to keep our clients informed as well as to ascertain their reactions to the trial. Sometimes we would be joined by Harold's wife, Betty, as well as my father, Sam[5].

I asked Michelle what she thought of the testimony of Dr. Harris.

"I felt it was another incidence of providence. Dennis and I felt this was the first incident where the pharmaceutical company deliberately hid information from the FDA. We thought to ourselves, how does this happen? But it does! It also proved to us and made us more furious, that they didn't even take Dr. Harris serious—poo-poo'd him. We asked ourselves, if they ignored this doctor, how many others did they ignore."

"Michelle and Dennis, tell me what you both thought about Dr. McCleery's testimony?"

Michelle said, "We had no idea the industry corruption ran so deep. Especially the testimony about the printed pamphlets that were never submitted to the FDA for approval—how come they get away with it? How inept our FDA really is—it's like the tail wagging the dog! We're amazed at the corruption disclosed today and feel good that we're doing the right thing."

---

5   My father had an opportunity only for an 8th grade education, when his father died and he had to go to work to help support the family of six. His dream growing up, however, was to be a lawyer. He had a brilliant mind and would watch almost every major case I tried into his eighties. His observations on the effect of witnesses on the jury was very helpful.

Michelle related how Dennis and she, "were in complete agreement that we had a big fight on our hands. Dr. Ley's testimony made us feel good because of his testimony that the FDA was intimidated by Big Pharma, and that intimidation was so terribly wrong. They had to have broken laws to do that—hide information from the FDA."

I informed them that the next witness would be among the most critical to the case. Despite hearing evidence from FDA officials, including the commissioner himself, that the "Pill" does cause blood clotting disorders in some women, and further that the industry deliberately attempted to conceal and create confusion on the causation issue, the main question in the jury's mind had not yet been addressed. Did the "Pill" cause Michelle's blindness? This primary issue would be addressed by the opinion testimony of Jerome Bettman, M.D. We hoped he would be our star witness who would cement causation between the "Pill" and her blindness specifically.

I was referred to Dr. Bettman by the nationally prominent pharmacologist I had retained as a consultant, but who, himself, refused to testify to avoid jeopardizing his position as the head of the Department of Pharmacology at a major U.S. university medical school.

CHAPTER 8
THE TRUTH UNFOLDS

JEROME BETTMAN, M.D.

As we entered the courthouse, meeting up with Dr. Bettman, he asked, "How do you think the case is progressing so far?"

"I believe the testimony we've been able to introduce has been exceptionally powerful in establishing evidence that there is general causation that the 'Pill' does cause thrombosis in some women. So, your testimony will be a logical sequence in connecting this to Michelle, personally."

"Good," Dr. Bettman said as we entered the courtroom.

We were surprised to find so many spectators waiting for trial to begin. Marion was with his team of lawyers at counsel table as the bailiff gave his usual announcement that Judge Allen would be taking the bench. Judge Allen took his seat and asked, "Counsel, do you have any matters you need to discuss outside the presence of the jury?"

"No, your Honor," Marion and I responded in unison.

Judge Allen turned to the bailiff, "Bailiff, bring in the jury."

Following the morning greetings, he looked at me saying, "Counsel, call your next witness."

"Your Honor, the Plaintiffs will call Dr. Jerome Bettman, to the stand." As I motioned Dr. Bettman toward the witness stand, with his briefcase in hand he confidently walked past the jury taking the witness chair as though it was his daily experience. The jury seemed focused on this short, elderly man with coke bottle glasses and a professorial appearance.

"Dr. Bettman, would you please detail for the jury, your medical background?"

"I am a board-certified California licensed ophthalmologist. I have been on the faculty of Stanford Medical School since 1937. I am now Emeritus clinical professor in ophthalmology at Stanford Medical School and a regular clinical professor at the University of California Medical School in San Francisco. I've been the chief of ophthalmology at Stanford Medical School, and for twenty-five years I have been on the faculty of the American Academy of Ophthalmology. For many years I have been involved in research on vascular disorders of the eye, edited a book on the subject, and have published over seventy-two articles dealing with the eye, many concerning vascular problems."

I interrupted. "Doctor, is thrombosis a vascular disorder within your area of expertise?"

"Yes, it is."

"Doctor, please continue with your medical background."

"I served as an associate examiner of the American Board of Ophthalmology. I am also a committee member of the National Institute of Health in the eye study section, determining what research grants in ophthalmology should be given within the United States, to whom, and how a proper study should be conducted. I've practiced ophthalmology for many years at various hospitals, including Stanford University Hospital, in Palo Alto, California, Children's Hospital, Mount Zion Hospital, and the University of California Hospital, all in San Francisco. For quite some period of time, I have testified before the FDA and served as their advisor on ophthalmic prescription drugs."

Demonstrating his balance of experience as well as lack of bias, Dr. Bettman went on to say he also represented a number of pharmaceutical companies and their problems at the FDA. However, he had never before testified in a "Pill" case, which added even more to his credibility. After hearing his impressive background, not one person in the courtroom should have questioned his competency and lack of bias.

Dr. Bettman explained to the jury that in the formulation of his opinion in this case, he reviewed all of Michelle's medical records, the depositions that had been taken of Michelle's treating doctors, specifically naming Drs. Kosmin, Noyes, Sogg, and Finkel, as well as a doctor for the Defense, Dr. Ostler. He explained how he reviewed adverse reaction cases of women on the "Pill," particularly those dealing with eye complications.

Dr. Bettman explained Michelle's blindness was permanent, total and irreversible as a result of atrophy of the optic nerve in each eye, ". . . due to a disturbance in the circulation of blood in the optic nerve and surrounding areas . . . caused by a block in the so-called venous return, that is, the veins that drain the blood away from the area have been stopped up by clots, by thrombi as they call it . . ." He described how this was caused by the "Pill" in combination with Type B blood and a blood infection. As a specialist in vascular problems of the eye, he was knowledgeable and convinced of the fact that *"The 'Pill' increases the chance of clotting by a very significant amount."*

As he described the anatomy involved, he explained the optic nerve enters from the back of the eye, into the skull and joins the other optic nerve at the optic chiasm. A number of veins drain the area, including the superior and inferior ophthalmic veins, into a pool of blood called the cavernous sinus. The blockage of drainage would have occurred in a number of places causing blindness. Then leaving the witness chair, this seasoned medical professor stepped down to a chalkboard on the nearby wall and placed numbers on the board as he testified.

He continued, ". . .conceding that the 'Pill' obviously does not cause clotting in everyone who takes it . . . but . . . there is a predisposed group of individuals who are more likely to clot than others and there are a number of factors that predispose towards further clotting. Now, if you want me to continue among those factors, well, in Mrs. Ahearn's case her blood type, for one thing, makes her more likely to clot than other types. She, as I recall, is Type B and Type B is approximately three times as likely to clot as Type O. Now, in addition to that, she was on the 'Pill' which makes her approximately, depending upon whose series you want to accept, makes her from about four-and-a-half to nine times as likely to clot as somebody who isn't on it. She apparently had a streptococcal invasion of some sort. This would likewise make her more likely to clot."

He repeatedly indicated and emphasized that the selected numbers were arbitrary and not intended as exact figures. Referring to the strep infection number, he testified:

"Nobody has demonstrated precisely how much more likely this makes her to clot, let's say this makes her another, just to pick a figure, four times. I don't know. Nobody knows, but this would then make her what is my arithmetic, thirty times as much likely to clot as if she were normal. Now, if you take away this strep factor, she is still eighteen times as likely. Now, you can debate how much streptococcal infection she had, but you can't debate the fact that she was on the 'Pill' and so this factor remains, this factor remains [indicating] so she is eighteen times as likely to clot as the person who was not on the 'Pill' and wasn't Type B with or without the strep. Put the strep in the picture and she is even more likely."

The point Dr. Bettman was attempting to explain was that a synergistic relationship occurred when clotting factors were combined. He then wrote down the mathematical formula he was attempting to explain. Although he wrote specific figures on the chalkboard, his testimony clearly demonstrated they were meant to be demonstrative of an accumulative effect, and not mathematically exact.

". . . The fact is that she was having significantly more likelihood to thrombose because of the combination of the 'Pill' and the blood type."

"Thank you, Doctor. Does it make any difference whether the infection came first before she thrombosed or after she thrombosed, in your opinion, as to the cause of the ultimate blindness?"

Dr. Bettman replied, "Here is a woman who is at greater risk because of the 'Pill' because of her blood type. Obviously, something had to push her over. In this case it could well have been the infection. Obviously, not every woman on the 'Pill' is going to develop thrombi or no one may be taking the 'Pill,' but the fact is that in a person who had this increased hazard because of the 'Pill' and blood type, then something came along that made her coagulate [thrombose], made her more likely to coagulate and whether she coagulated first because of the 'Pill' and then got an infection or had the infection and had already, of course, been taking the 'Pill' and coagulated on that account, I don't think is terribly important. The fact is that she, as I said before, is coagulated, is more likely to because she was on the 'Pill' and B blood type and she had something else in the picture that pushed her over that, lighted her keg of dynamite. And that, I suppose, was the strep infection or could have been."

Addressing the Defense theory, that the sole cause of Michelle's blindness was orbital cellulitis (a strep infection in the soft tissue of the face around the cheek and orbit of the eye), I asked Dr. Bettman the following, "Doctor, in your opinion is it very likely that a woman such as Michelle who was *not* on the 'Pill' would experience total complete bilateral blindness from a strep infection whether it be cellulitis or pharyngitis?"

"No, I should say not."

"Have you seen cases of orbital cellulitis?"

"Yes, I have seen a good many cases of orbital cellulitis."

"Have you ever seen a case of orbital cellulitis that resulted in total permanent bilateral blindness?"

"Not bilateral, no, never. I have never seen one and furthermore, I don't know of anyone else that did see one."

"What makes the difference in Michelle's case, Doctor?"

"Well, again it is something unusual about her and I think that unusual factor was the 'Pill.'"

Thus, the key factual issue on causation became what caused the increased risk in someone already predisposed. Dr. Bettman clearly was convinced that the key factor was the "Pill," and infection alone did not, and could not, cause the thrombosis and ultimate blindness.

On cross-examination, the Defense could not weaken the strength of his testimony or create any doubt in his opinions. They attempted to play a numbers game with Dr. Bettman by attempting to tie him down to an exact multiple he was contending each factor played. However, that was nothing more than a waste of time. Dr. Bettman was very clear that he was utilizing multiples in the generic sense and that it would be impossible for anyone to come up with a precise number.

In that Dr. Bettman's qualifications were unimpeachable, they couldn't create any gains in that area with the jury. He had testified on direct examination of a conversation he had in the hallway of a hospital with Dr. Sogg, Michelle's treating neuro-ophthalmologist, wherein Dr. Bettman contended that Dr. Sogg admitted the possibility of the "Pill" as a cause given Dr. Bettman's scenario of events. The Defense cross-examined him particularly on this issue which accomplished little.

The Defense then chose the following tactic. They dropped the subject and chose to attack Dr. Bettman's credibility as to this conversation later in the trial when they presented Dr. Sogg as part of the Defense case. Dr. Sogg denied he made the admission that he agreed with Dr. Bettman's theory as being correct.

Dr. Bettman's testimony ended the trial day. The Court recessed and instructed the jury to return at 9 a.m. the next morning. Harold, Michelle, Dennis and I left together, as usual, and met up with Dr. Bettman waiting for the elevator.

Dr. Bettman turned to Michelle and told her, "Michelle, the optic nerve is the most susceptible in the body. It was a forgone conclusion that after five minutes from the blood clots cutting the circulation off, you would have been blind." He wished her well as he left the courthouse.

Michelle turned to us. "Dr. Bettman's testimony, demeanor, confidence and the way he testified indicated he was very knowledgeable. You had to believe what he said."

Dennis jumped in, "This man knew what he was talking about. Straight forward, honest testimony."

Both added they felt very good after his testimony. Harold and I agreed with them and hoped the jury saw him that way as well. Harold commented that the jury was really focused on Dr. Bettman and their facial expressions indicated they appeared to accept his testimony. I added that his lifetime skills as a professor seemed to make the jury look at Dr. Bettman as a teacher and his tutorial approach definitely put them in a classroom environment. We parted for the day to return to my office to prepare the witness, Dr. Altshuler, for the next morning, who was flying in from his home in Colorado.

JOHN ALTSHULER, M.D.

Dr. Altshuler, was a highly respected hematologist and a personal friend of Harold Williams. When we initially asked him to review

Michelle's records and testify, if he felt the case was meritorious, he graciously agreed despite his own heavy personal practice. I felt it would be critical to present testimony from a hematologist since that specialty required a thorough understanding of the causes of blood clotting. Dr. Altshuler's credentials, in my opinion, rendered him extraordinarily competent to express an opinion on causation in Michelle's case specifically.

Harold and I met Dr. Altshuler for breakfast at his hotel the next morning and further discussed his upcoming trial testimony. Dr. Altshuler, having the experience of testifying in a few oral contraceptive cases, was confident of his opinions on the issues involved. As we entered the courtroom, I was somewhat surprised to again observe a significant number of spectators awaiting the trial day to begin. The judge quickly came out and had the jury called in.

He requested me to present my next witness.

"Your Honor, the Plaintiffs call Dr. John Altshuler to the stand as their next witness."

Dr. Altshuler testified to his qualifications, "I am licensed to practice medicine in California and Colorado, double board-certified in anatomic and clinical pathology since 1965 and immunohematology since 1973. I had two post doctorate fellowship years at Yale Medical Center in the field of clinical pathology and coagulation hematology, the latter concentrating on clotting and bleeding disorders and mechanisms in the laboratory and in patients. I am currently the professor in Clotting and Bleeding Disorders at the University of Colorado Medical School Hospital and regularly lecture other specialties on the clotting mechanism. My clinical practice since 1965 has been *exclusively* physician referrals of bleeding and clotting disorders. My publications in the medical literature dealt primarily with *drug related coagulation problems*, including the 'Pill.'"

His qualifications, learning and clinical experience in dealing with clotting problems, especially drug related, were unmatched by any other medical witness in the entire case presented by either side.

"Dr. Altshuler, do you have an opinion as to whether the 'Pill' causes blood clotting in some women?"

"Yes, it certainly does."

"What is the basis of that opinion?"

"My opinion is that the 'Pill' causes clotting and I'm primarily relying on my own clinical experience and not merely medical literature or laboratory work. I have treated two cases of cavernous sinus thrombosis caused by the 'Pill.' The estrogen component of the 'Pill' is the primary cause of clotting and that estrogen therapy has been used by some physicians for years to treat bleeders. Challenge and response cases comprise the most convincing evidence. I saw a case of a husband who mistakenly took his wife's oral contraceptive and developed massive brain thrombosis."

He emphasized the importance of the challenge and response cases which he had read in Dr. Ley's deposition. Dr. Altshuler had thoroughly studied the medical records and Michelle's medical history. He testified that his opinions took into consideration all the significant facts, circumstances, and symptoms preceding hospitalization as they were established in the record by lay witnesses and Dr. Gossack's records.

He explained, from a clotting expert's viewpoint, that the logical sequence of events in the mechanism of blindness in Michelle was consistent with the entire record of evidence, including hospital records. He acknowledged the septicemia and infection, but logically pointed out that Michelle's clinical course would suggest it was a secondary event in that the systemic component of infection—high fever, fast heart rate, chills and shock—were not present and did not develop until the following day. Thrombosis itself, he explained, creates a medium of bacterial growth which would substantiate the thrombosis developing before the infection. In other words, blood clotting could have preceded the strep infection in Michelle.

"The pterygoid plexus and ophthalmic veins are the region where the thrombosis developed. The unusual site of thrombosis in Michelle [the pterygoid plexus] is consistent with the "unusual sites" where thrombosis occurs in 'Pill' users as reported in the literature and in my personal, medical experience."

His testimony to predisposition created by the "Pill" became clear when he stated she was, ". . . set up, a sitting duck, that has already been primed with birth control or estrogen . . . medication that already makes them prey to any complications, whether it be sepsis [infection], whether it be injury, whether it be shock, no matter what the insult is . . ." He explained that for those reasons, surgeons take their patients off the "Pill" for some period of time prior to surgery.

The testimony of Dr. Altshuler was persuasive to the jury as demonstrated by the questions several jurors addressed to him at the end of his testimony.

A juror questioned, "I would like to ask you if your thesis of sequence of events supporting thrombosis diagnosis in Michelle's case was not the basis for your two plusses on clinical designation.

And if I am right in my memory of your previous testimony, that you based that thesis on Dr. Gossack's medical record of her case equally at least as any of the other records because he was the one that saw her before the hospital."

Dr. Altshuler's sincerity and objectivity was particularly communicated in the following response:

"... I am not so primed in my own mind that I will look at every thrombotic case that comes along that has the 'Pill' attached to it and jump to the conclusion that that is the cause. I have seen many cases . . . that I have been approached about and I just don't think it's tenable . . . Now, I don't have any question in this case what's happened. I feel very strongly, as you have gathered of course. I think the clinical story from beginning to end taking into account all the records, Dr. Gossack, Dr. Kosmin, Dr. Lippe—I don't know if I have missed anyone—Dr. Brooks, I believe the ENT man, I have taken all of them into account in the clinical story. I'm not trying to double plus on the clinical side here. If one were to just add up the laboratory studies, the clinical course, the fact that she was on medicine [oral contraceptive], the fact that she was really thrown over the balance with hypercoagulable status due to medication [oral contraceptive], it just adds up to me."

He re-emphasized in great detail the "sitting duck" concept as to the role of the "Pill" when a woman is subjected to a variety of traumas. This testimony was, of course, consistent with the opinion of Dr. Bettman.

∽

Of particular relevance to the lack of warnings by the industry, a juror asked the following question: "In your opinion, would it be more difficult for a specialist such as a neurosurgeon or an ENT man or any other specialty that would not normally prescribe an oral contraceptive to get the information about the general studies on oral contraceptives and the possible cause and effect relationship or even the statistically significant association? What I am saying is, you as a specialist, if you want information about this drug and you think it might be related to a case, do you pick up the PDR? Do you have a package insert that's been provided to you automatically or do you go to your journals?"

Dr. Altshuler responded.

". . . the patients I see are all very sick and complicated and they take a lot of time and I have the time to sit down and read the articles, but a doctor that sees thirty people a day, in no way can he go to the library sit down and do it, he just can't do it, there is not enough time. The demands are too great. You have got to rely on the pharmaceutical companies to provide the information and to tell you 'yes, we have done this work and we have shown clearly that there is a cause and effect relationship between thrombosis and the 'Pill.'' And that's going to alert the physician to say 'gee, do I want to take that risk?' . . . I am talking about the average practicing physician . . . does not have the time to go out and read the Vessey and Doll reports and this and that and this comprehensive article here, they just can't do it . . . He has got to rely on what he is told by the package insert and the detail man that comes around to give you the drug."

Cross-examination of Dr. Altshuler accomplished little for the Defense. Rather it provided further opportunity for him to explain in even greater medical detail, in clear language to a lay jury, the basis for his strong position on the mechanism of how the

"Pill" contributed to Michelle's blindness. As a specialist in blood clotting, he was the wrong witness to expect to create doubt on a medical issue within the core of his specialty.

At dinner that evening, I asked Michelle her impression of Dr. Altshuler's testimony.

"Wow! I felt like a pincushion as I listened to his explanation of what happened to me. I got hit from all different directions and I didn't have a chance to escape severe consequences." She went on to discuss how important she felt his testimony was. "He provided further clinical proof that the 'Pill' caused my blood to clot."

I left dinner early so I could prepare my next witness, Dr. Leissring, by telephone that evening. He resided in Santa Rosa, California.

JOHN LEISSRING, M.D.

Dr. Leissring was a past client and a friend of mine for some years back. I was always impressed with his scholarly approach to medicine and specifically his ability to properly diagnose an illness as well as its cause.

Dr. Leissring drove to San Jose early the next morning and met me at my office where together with Harold, we drove to the courthouse as we discussed his pending testimony. I filled Dr. Leissring in on the witnesses that had testified so far. Hearing this, he felt even more comfortable about testifying, realizing his opinion on the "Pill" would corroborate prior testimony.

Judge Allen instructed me to call my next witness.

"Your Honor, Plaintiffs would call Dr. John Leissring to the stand as our next witness."

Dr. Leissring walked up to the witness stand, a young, attractive, tall, athletic looking physician, a real contrast to previous witnesses.

He testified to the following credentials: board-certified in pathology, a graduate of the University of Wisconsin Medical School, had his internship and five years of general practice in the U.S. Navy, then four years of pathology at Stanford with six years of pathology practice at the time of trial, some of which was at O'Connor Hospital Pathology Department in San Jose (where Michelle was treated) and hospitals in Santa Rosa, California. He further attained a master's degree in anatomy, which was unusual. His current practice of pathology consisted of the diagnostic aspects of medical practice. His expertise was in laboratory testing, tissue diagnosis, examination of fluids taken from the body, and consultative type of practice in which ". . . physicians who are having difficulty making certain diagnoses come to our practice for aid in diagnosis." He has been involved in autopsy toxicology as well as the study of blood coagulation problems in living people "by such simple things as aspirin and antibiotics."

Dr. Leissring had never testified in a "Pill" case. He reviewed Michelle's medical chart in a manner similar to that used in his daily practice as a consultant to treating physicians and during clinical pathologic conferences on specific patients. He compared his findings in the medical literature with his experience and could not find any support in the literature for streptococcal disease being the primary event in the cause of bilateral blindness. His research disclosed cases "similar" to Michelle's, particularly in the French and German medical literature in which the "Pill" was the primary cause. He analyzed the evidence of strep infection from a pathologist's viewpoint, emphasizing the lack of positive evidence of its existence anywhere in Michelle other than her blood stream.

"The classic results of cellulitis are to be able to see the organisms directly by just smearing them on a slide and staining for them, and not only did this not occur, but they were not able to culture organisms from this fluid and this was prior to having received any antibiotics . . . The diagnosis is only made on the basis of presence of organisms in the infected tissue and none were found [in Michelle]."

"High fever, shaking chills, and other severe symptoms always accompany a septicemia from strep." He concluded, "And in the absence of any other evidence of septic embolization, I would doubt that this so-called bacteremia or septicemia was significant."

He viewed the thrombosis as beginning "in a position which was dually draining both the brain and the facial tissues," and noted that one of the treating doctors, Dr. Brooks (ENT), dictated his postoperative diagnosis of *cavernous sinus thrombosis* after Michelle was discharged from the hospital and Dr. Brooks had available to him her entire hospital record. Dr. Leissring's analysis, as a pathologist, of the laboratory findings and treating physicians' notes reported in the records all supported thrombosis primary and infection as secondary.

Cross-examination of Dr. Leissring was uneventful and accomplished little, if anything for the Defense. Marion, in the usual approach to create a suspicion of bias in an opposition expert witness, asked "Dr. Leissring, how much are you being paid in this case?"

"I am acting as a friend of the Court. I may not charge anything," Dr. Leissring offered. In fact, he refused to accept any payment for his time in testifying in this case. Marion failed to ask what would have been the killer follow-up question. "Are you a friend of Sal Liccardo?" to which Jack would have had to respond affirmatively.

During a break, I asked Michelle and Dennis for their reaction to Dr. Leissring.

Michelle said excitedly, "When he was asked how much he was going to be paid, and he answered, "I'm here at the service of the Court,' I wanted to jump up and down and shout 'hurray for the good guys!' It felt like the air was sucked out of the Defense side of the room."

Dennis asked, "Who's next?"

Harold responded, "The next witness is my good friend, Dr. Overton," whom we had prepared the evening before.

MARTIN OVERTON, M.D.

Dr. Overton was a neurosurgeon from Fort Worth, Texas. Harold had worked with him in several prior "Pill" cases which were unsuccessful, however, he did feel that Dr. Overton would be ideal for the *Ahearn* case.

He was right. We returned from the break and Judge Allen asked me to present my next witness.

"Your Honor, Plaintiffs call Dr. Martin Overton to the stand."

After reviewing his formal medical educational background, he described his specialization in neurosurgery since 1962, including his U.S. Air Force experience as Chief of Neurosurgery at Travis Air force base in California, as well as consultant to the California Prison System. He returned to private practice in Fort Worth, Texas in 1968. He explained that thrombosis problems within the head and skull were a major area of his practice and interest. He had lectured OB-GYNs on oral contraceptive complications and had testified in previous "Pill" cases against the pharmaceutical companies, but not Johnson & Johnson.

Dr. Overton informed the jury that he had reviewed Michelle's complete medical records and the deposition of Dr. Kosmin, her initial treating doctor when she entered the hospital. He further conducted a personal consultation with Michelle.

"Doctor, do you have an opinion as to whether Ortho-Novum was a substantial factor in causing Michelle's blindness?"

With his Texas flair and accent he replied, "Yes, her blindness resulted from the oral contraceptive through a thrombosis mechanism causing venous backup creating increased intra cranial pressure. This intra cranial pressure explained her severe headache at the onset of her illness. Increased intra cranial pressure and venous backup reaches the head of the optic nerve through the dura track thereby resulting in optic atrophy [death of the cells in the optic nerve]."

"Doctor, do you have an opinion as to the role of infection in her case?"

"She did not have infectious meningitis [infection within the fluid in the brain and spinal column]. Infection was not the primary problem."

He concurred with the other Plaintiffs' experts, Dr. Leissring, pathologist, Dr. Altshuler, hematologist, and Dr. Bettmen, ophthalmologist, who had all testified that a *secondary* infection is possible when there is swelling of tissue as a result of vascular obstructions, such as thrombi. They each explained how an obstruction to the flow of blood in a vessel creates a pooling of blood and fluids, thereby providing an excellent medium for the growth of bacteria, particularly infectious organisms. The swelling of tissue allows external or surface bacteria to permeate through the soft tissue in the area, thereby setting up an infected area.

He added, "Most significantly, Michelle's medical records confirm that blood cultures identifying strep bacteria had not been taken until after swelling had begun."

Then he dropped a bomb on Ortho.

I asked, "Doctor, have you had any experience with Ortho Pharmaceutical Company in the past?"

He told his story.

"In 1967 [two years before Michelle's blindness], I personally reported a stroke case which I believed was caused by the 'Pill' to Ortho. I was told by Ortho, "You are on the wrong track, doctor. Don't go on pursuing this. I subsequently learned that Ortho misrepresented to the FDA that my patient had recovered when reporting this adverse reaction case. In fact, she was paralyzed on one side of her body, unable to speak or to understand."

Dr. Overton went on to describe to the jury many other cases of stroke which he believed were caused by the "Pill" as the treating physician, including three challenge and response cases.

Dr. Overton accused Ortho of "suppressing information" in the following testimony:

". . . there is good evidence that the 'Pill' increases the incidence of stroke that the company did not put it or did not make it available in any way for the physician at a time when it was available. They did not put out information saying this or any kind of a warning as to cause and effect through the detail men, into the Physicians' Desk Reference, into the package insert, or anywhere.

They did not put that information out for us and that's why the value of a prepared mind issues its head here."

In brief, his testimony to this jury painted a clear picture of "commercial callousness," and a "conscious disregard of safety" toward women taking the "Pill" by Ortho and other "Pill" manufacturers.

Marion's cross-examination of Dr. Overton was the most rigorous and vicious so far in the trial. Ortho's counsel attacked his character head on attempting to paint him as a paid prostitute who makes a fortune testifying in "Pill" cases. Over my repeated objections, overruled by Judge Allen, Ortho's counsel harped upon a substantial consultation fee Dr. Overton had received in another past "Pill" case in which he had testified as an expert, calling it excessive. The only relationship between that case and this involved contentions that the "Pill" caused thrombosis, yet Ortho's counsel never asked him even once what his fee was in the *Ahearn* case! That would have been a relevant question to determine bias of the witness. Fearing stepping into the same trap as they did with Dr. Leissring, they feared his answer might be zero. The Defense was not going to make that mistake again.

However, the failure of the Court to sustain my objections to this irrelevant testimony concerning what happened in some other case was inexcusable in my mind, further supporting my earlier suspicion of judicial bias. The belligerency, hostility, and agitation of the Defense counsel in its blatant attack upon this witness' integrity was inexcusable, yet despite repeated requests to Judge Allen, I was overruled, and the hostile questioning was allowed to continue. Even the witness himself, Dr. Overton, felt compelled under these embarrassing circumstances to plead for some civility, decency, and gentlemanly conduct from the Defense, all to no avail. The ultimate effect of this tactic by Ortho upon the jury was fast becoming one of our major concerns.

The refusal of Judge Allen to stop the hostility, created against a primary Plaintiff's expert witness, his constant critical tone when he questioned Plaintiffs' experts, together with his repeated biased comments in the presence of the jury from the beginning of trial worried me. It caused me to fear the jury was being unfairly swayed to the favor of the Defense. Jurors typically look up to the trial judge and take seriously every word he/she utters, as well as the rulings made. The apparent bias of the judge by this point of the trial appeared to me to be overwhelming.

Harold shared my feelings on this issue. Based on prior discussions, I knew he was in full agreement with me that we take the risk of losing this jury by making a motion for mistrial, even though we felt comfortable that overall it was a good jury for us.

I therefore felt compelled to do something I had never done before, nor since, in a trial. I requested the Court that we be allowed to recess and go into chambers with a court reporter so I could make a motion. Judge Allen agreed, dismissing the jury for the rest of the day, and moved the proceedings into his chambers away from public view. The judge clearly anticipated the nature of my motion.

"Your Honor, I am sorry I have to do this, but I am compelled to move for a mistrial based upon a clear bias against our case exhibited by this Court in the presence of the jury that is certain to influence them against the Plaintiffs." I then cited for the record the multiple comments and rulings that he had made in the presence of the jury indicating, in my mind, a clear bias in the Defense's favor and against the Plaintiffs.

Marion, of course, opposed our motion denying there was any bias in anything that Judge Allen had said or done. We felt confident he would deny the motion, but it was critical that we get his bias on the record in the event of an appeal. Such procedure would strengthen an argument on appeal that the jury was wrongfully influenced by the conduct of the judge, if it were a Defense verdict.

Judge Allen calmly gave me a strange smile as he professionally denied my motion, as I expected. For roughly three days thereafter, the judge withheld his offensive comments indicating bias while in the jury's presence, only to fall back on his same old pattern for the remainder of the trial.

Following this extensive motion, the Court recessed until the next morning. We explained to Michele and Dennis what had occurred in chambers, and why we had to do it at that time to preserve the record on appeal. Both agreed fully with what we had done because they, too, were outraged by the conduct allowed by the Court on cross-examination by Dr. Overton, but expressed some anxiety at what reaction the Judge might have towards us the next day and during the rest of the trial.

J. RAY VAN METER, M.D.

Harold and I rushed back to my office to take advantage of the available time to hopefully prepare our next witness in person. I phoned Dr. Van Meter and asked if he could make time for us if we came to his office. He said he would work in the time. We drove to Palo Alto, I introduced Harold to Dr. Van Meter since they had never met, and we reviewed his anticipated testimony with him.

Knowing from past defense expert depositions that their key defense would claim that the sole cause of Michelle's blindness was infection and not thrombosis, I retained Dr. Van Meter because of his very unusual experience with infection in the cavernous sinus and the skull. He was a neurologist with whom I had worked with in other cases.

The next morning Harold and I met up with Dr. Van Meter at the courthouse. We walked into Judge Allen's courtroom uneasy as to what to expect following my motion yesterday accusing him of bias. When he entered the courtroom, to my pleasant surprise, Judge Allen was unusually cordial and respectful toward everyone, including me.

"You may call your next witness, counsel."

"Your Honor, the Plaintiffs will call Dr. Van Meter to the stand."

Old and stern in appearance, Dr. Van Meter slowly made his way to the witness stand. He had testified many times in Santa Clara County courts, both as a neurologist and psychiatrist, and was probably recognized by Judge Allen as testifying in his Court in the past.

"Doctor, would you please provide us with your medical background and experience?"

"I am double board-certified in neurology and psychiatry, but I practice chiefly in the field of neurology. I taught as a professor of neurology at the University of Pennsylvania from 1933-1937, and at Temple University graduate school from 1937-1942. I then served in the armed forces during WWII practicing neurology until 1946, when I joined the faculty of the University of California

Medical School for the next twenty-one years. I am presently an emeritus professor of neurology at that institution."

To make it easier for the jury to understand, Dr. Van Meter created a time flow chart to illustrate the significance of symptoms and findings obtained from Michelle's medical records. He then demonstrated the significance of the order of medical observations such as temperature, swelling, and laboratory findings. The time chart negated infection as the primary cause, but rather thrombosis of the pterygoid plexus and cavernous sinus as the mechanism of blindness, and the "Pill" as its cause.

His advanced age gave him an unusual persuasive advantage as being the only physician in the case who had extensive experience in the pre-antibiotic age, while practicing in three large metropolitan hospitals in the East, a time when cavernous sinus thrombosis was more commonly seen. He described details of these experiences.

He explained, "The presence of strep bacteria in the blood, as found in Michelle, can occur *without severe septicemia*—a life threatening infection. If she had severe septicemia from strep, a source would have been found, such as an abscess or infection in the bladder, kidney or elsewhere on her body. No such signs of a serious infection were ever found in Michelle."

Cross-examination of Dr. Van Meter was brief and uneventful. Due to his vast pre-antibiotic specific experience there was little Marion could cross-examine him on effectively.

During both direct and cross-examination of Dr. Van Meter, Judge Allen was quite respectful and unbiased with his comments. He then excused the jurors for the usual morning recess.

I went over to Michele and Dennis.

"Do you feel better about Judge Allen now?"

Both reserved making any comment, then Michele offered, "After hearing Dr. Van Meter's testimony it's like we're building one brick on top of the other, making it hard for the Defense to knock down our case."

LARRY GOSSACK, M.D.

The next witness lined up for that morning was Dr. Gossack, Michelle's OB-GYN. He had arrived during the prior testimony and was sitting in the back of the spectators' section. At the break Michelle, Dennis and I went back to engage him. He greeted Michelle warmly as they talked socially for a few moments. I had met with Dr. Gossack at his office before the trial began to prepare him for his testimony. He had been cooperative with me and understood his primary role was to lay out the medical history and facts related to Michelle and the case for the jury. He appeared confident and most willing to be of help. His natural demeanor was one of a gentle, caring personal physician and he carried that demeanor onto the witness stand.

As Michelle's treating OB-GYN for several years and the physician involved at the very beginning of her illness, Dr. Gossack's testimony was crucial. He was the only physician to have seen Michelle during her initial onset of illness.

"You may call your next witness."

"Thank you, your Honor, the Plaintiffs call Dr. Larry Gossack to the stand."

"Doctor, please describe your medical background for the jury?"

"I am board-certified in obstetrics and gynecology. I taught Obstetrics and Gynecology at Northwestern University Medical School, as well as hospital programs in the San Jose area. I have been in private practice in San Jose for over twenty years."

"You are Michell's personal physician and OB-GYN?"

"Michelle has been my patient for general health and OB-GYN care for over seven years and continues to today."

"Doctor, are you the only physician who examined Michelle before her illness resulting in her blindness?"

"Yes, I saw her and gave her a thorough examination on February 16, 1969, before her admission to the Hospital that evening. The examination took place between 2:00 p.m. and 2:30 p.m. that afternoon."

"Did you find any evidence whatsoever of infection?"

"No. My exam completely negated any medical evidence whatsoever of an infectious presence or process. She had no sore throat, no redness, swelling or tenderness in any area of her throat, eyes, face, ears, lymph nodes, nor any observations of pus or exudate. I took her temperature and it was *normal*. I was surprised by that."

Temperature was testified to by every other expert, as an "absolute necessity" in diagnosing a strep infection.

He went on, "The only symptom present at that time was a one-sided headache and the only sign was tenderness in the jugular vein area of her neck. Upon having her hospitalized, I referred her to a neurosurgeon, Dr. Lippe, for further consultation and follow-up confirming that the headache was the only sign or symptom that I could determine at that time."

Although Dr. Gossack expressed no opinion as to the cause of Michelle's blindness, which he considered beyond his expertise, his testimony clearly negated infection as an initial cause and confirmed physical findings consistent with thrombosis of the pterygoid plexis in the form of tenderness at that general location. His initial physical examination provided a sound medical basis for the ultimate opinions of the other Plaintiffs' experts who testified that *thrombosis* and *not* infection was the major player in Michelle's illness.

Dr. Gossack's testimony provided the answer to another critical issue in the case. If Ortho had warned that the "Pill" had a *cause and effect* relationship with thrombosis, and such warning had reached Dr. Gossack and Michelle, would Michelle have taken the "Pill" anyway? Michelle testified in her deposition that she would not have taken the "Pill" if she had known the risks. Dr. Gossack clearly stated that had cause and effect information been clearly stated and made available to him, "I would have warned Michelle and probably not have prescribed the 'Pill' for her."

Dr. Gossack identified Thomas Preston as the Ortho representative that would call upon him periodically during the two years he was prescribing the "Pill" to Michelle.

"Did Mr. Preston ever tell you of any adverse reaction reports from other physicians relating the 'Pill" to thrombosis?"

"No."

"Did Mr. Preston ever tell you of any ongoing study in Great Britain suggesting a cause and effect relationship between the 'Pill' and thrombosis?"

"No."

He testified that Mr. Preston never told him of any reported cases of the "Pill" causing thrombosis in anyone, nor of any study indicating a possible causal relationship between the "Pill" and thromboembolic disease. Mr. Preston had provided the patient booklets displayed in Dr. Gossack's waiting room, describing the benefits and emphasizing the safety of the "Pill," without any warnings of thrombosis risks. Michelle had picked up and read one of these Ortho booklets.

Dr. Gossack's credibility and integrity came through firmly in his testimony. Marion's cross-examination attempted to point out ways Dr. Gossack could have missed signs of infection but failed. Dr. Gossack's credibility remained intact.

Judge Allen then extensively and unfairly cross-examined Dr. Gossack as to whether he would prescribe the "Pill" *after* the trial, as well as what kind of warning he would give patients *after* the trial. A sample of his questioning was as follows:

"Well, did you know in 1967 that the 'Pill' can cause clots?"

"You were aware of that in 1967?"

"What does that mean, not proven or disproven?"

"Does that mean you disregard it?"

"What did you wonder?"

"Is this something you ignore or something you look out for?"

"You mean in the patients or in the literature?"

"Doctor, did you know this lady was on the 'Pill'?"

"When she came in to see you with a headache, didn't you know she was on the 'Pill'?"

"You knew about the British studies, didn't you?"

"Weren't you aware of these British publications?"

"I don't know what 'to any degree' means. Tell me what you did know."

"You still prescribe it, don't you?"

"You are going to prescribe it tomorrow, aren't you?"

"For a new patient you maybe never saw before?"

"You are now aware of this British article, right?"

"Well, what would you have done differently in 1968 than you are going to do tomorrow?"

"What are you going to tell this patient tomorrow?"

"I want to know what you are going to tell her as far as the risk of having a stroke is concerned?"

This was improper questioning by a trial judge in a jury case. At this point, Judge Allen clearly reverted back to his old pattern of displaying his bias to the jury. How could Dr. Gossack know in a vacuum what a particular patient might present by way of health factors for or against prescribing the "Pill?"

As we left the courthouse after his testimony, Michelle told me she felt sorry for Dr. Gossack. "He's been my doctor for eight years. He's a very good-hearted man and cares about his patients. I felt so bad seeing him up there because he felt really bad about what happened to me."

It always amazed me how Michelle would describe *seeing* people and things she really could not see at all. Obviously, everything would be visualized in her imagination, however, she couldn't have been more accurate in her description of Dr. Gossack on the stand. That was exactly how he came across in his testimony.

THOMAS PRESTON

The next day, we began testimony with the reading of Thomas Preston, the detail man for Ortho who I deposed in Puerto Rico in the winter of 1973. I requested Judge Allen to allow Harold to take the witness stand and read the answers while I read the questions. This would help the jury more easily follow the testimony. This approach reduces the boredom of the jury in having to listen to only one person read the deposition.

Harold read, "I was Ortho's 'detail man,' who called upon Dr. Gossack from 1965 through March 1969. A 'detail man' is a representative of a pharmaceutical manufacturer who calls upon a physician to inform him of the product. It was my job to emphasize only positive aspects about the 'Pill,' and never to discuss adverse effects other than as contained in the package insert or patient booklet. No warnings of thrombosis as a side effect were contained in such Ortho publications during that time period."

He continued, "Ortho *never* requested its detail men to encourage or solicit any adverse reaction reports from the physicians we called upon, nor to convey information on adverse reactions we received. We were not even to discuss with the physician the relationship between the "Pill" and thrombosis in *any* manner, regardless of the source of such information, whether adverse reaction reports or medical studies."

He further confirmed that no such discussions ever occurred with Dr. Gossack. Therefore, the warnings available to prescribing physicians, and particularly to Dr. Gossack, were whatever might be in the package insert or patient booklets—which were none at that time as to any serious side effects.

ALICE

Following the reading of Preston's deposition, we requested a recess before calling our next witness, Michelle's close friend, Alice. I met her in the courtroom during the break, and as with most lay witnesses, tried to get her to relax and reduce the natural stress and fear of taking the witness stand.

When we resumed after the break, I advised Judge Allen she would be our next witness. As she took the stand, I first had her identify herself as a good friend of Michelle. I then had her describe the events of the day she spent with Michelle immediately preceding her illness. Alice described her observations of Michelle as to her health before that day and during the time she was with Michelle. She denied observing any signs or symptoms of a cold, sore throat or fever in Michelle, as well as hearing any complaints as such from her. In short, she described Michelle as appearing to be in excellent health before and during that day. Her lay observations corroborated the medical testimony of Dr. Gossack that there were no signs of an infection within the few days leading up to her hospitalization. Alice's factual testimony left little room for cross-examination.

❦

Having completed our witnesses for the day, we packed up our files for the weekend. We asked Dennis and Michele if we could meet with them for dinner to discuss their upcoming testimony. They agreed and left.

Harold and I left the courthouse discussing a major issue at this juncture of the case. Had we presented enough witnesses and live testimony to convince the jury? Was this the right time to end our "case in chief" with the testimony of Dennis and Michelle? "Case in chief" is the technical legal term used to describe the total amount of evidence which a plaintiff must put on at the beginning of the trial to meet the burden of proof standard.

I preferred to place my clients on the stand last for several reasons. Having spent many days watching others testify, Dennis and Michele would be more comfortable with the rigid atmosphere of the courtroom and its strict procedures. Further, having heard the favorable, strong evidence in their case, they would realize the case is proven sufficiently such that the weight of convincing a jury no longer rested upon their testimony alone. Last, but not least, in this case I felt that Dennis and especially Michelle would be good witnesses with characteristic honesty and integrity that could only seal a conviction in the minds of the jury that the case was meritorious, and the Plaintiffs were worthy of a verdict.

Harold and I came to the same conclusion immediately. It was time to put closure to our case in chief by placing Dennis and Michelle on the stand. Even though there were three additional experts we had retained in the wings ready to testify, they would only be duplicative of what we had already presented. We also realized that Judge Allen could abruptly interfere with their testimony once he realized they were cumulative of evidence already presented. So, by ending now, we could avoid the potential situation that might make the jury think we were unnecessarily stretching out the trial on them. Juries never like that.

We met early that evening at our usual restaurant. I announced to Dennis that he would be our next witness, Michelle would follow and she would be the last witness. Both expressed their satisfaction with how strong of a case we had presented and felt confident that the jury so far was with them.

I then took each of them through the areas I would direct my questioning. I told them all they had to do was tell the truth—their story. Dennis commented, "This will be very emotional for me. I'll try to be brave, but I'm an emotional person."

Michelle reminded me, "Before the trial, you never intimated anything to me but to present the truth. I said to you, we have to get at the truth and only the truth. I am not walking into that courtroom with a cane and dark glasses. I don't want any sympathy to come into the verdict if it could be helped. I just want the truth!"

As we parted I repeated my advice to them not to worry about cross-examination. They would only be telling their true story, and Marion would know that from their previous depositions. Therefore, he would be gentle and respectful toward them on the stand, being the smart trial lawyer that he was. They were grateful for the preparation and left nervous, but eager to get it over with.

Dennis Ahearn

Monday morning, we greeted Dennis and Michelle at the courthouse. As we stepped into the elevator to get to Judge Allen's courtroom, I observed the anticipated nervousness in Dennis.

"Are you ready to take on Ortho?" I asked him hoping to lighten the mood and his stress.

"You bet," he said.

Judge Allen took the bench and asked, "Counsel, are you ready with your next witness?"

"Yes, your Honor. The Plaintiffs would like to call Dennis Ahearn to the stand."

I put Dennis on the stand to confirm Michelle's medical background and good health before this illness, the symptoms and observations he observed, and the order they occurred during the onset of the illness leading to the blindness. He was very clear on never observing any sign of infection such as fever, cough, complaints of sore throat and such. He described in great detail the whole ordeal from his observations as a lay person and her husband.

I asked Dennis how Michelle was adapting to a life of blindness from his observations. He described her tremendous courage following her blindness, how she undertakes her duties as a mother and wife, and the modifications he has created to help her. Where possible, he eliminated steps in their home, arranged furniture to help her avoid walking into things or being tripped by objects, etc. Very telling to the jury was his description of the effects of blindness on Michelle:

"She . . . has lost all of her independence as an individual to be able to function as a mother and a wife to me . . . She now struggles to achieve the simplest of household and motherly duties . . . She suffers embarrassment in such simple activities as dining in public . . . Boredom is a major problem for her . . . She has difficulty keeping track of the children as they run and play around the home. She's fearful of every ring of the doorbell or knock on the door. Unusual sounds that occur in the home would distress her and such."

Dennis was a credible and effective witness and no one in the courtroom could disbelieve a word he spoke. Testifying on Michelle's disability was a visible emotional strain on him that the jury could clearly observe. Marion wisely was gentle and politely cross-examined Dennis, as I expected. He only hit on a few points of no real consequence in the case.

Judge Allen then took over questioning Dennis in a cross-examination approach, somewhat rude and quite biased in my opinion, considering that I as his attorney could not object to questions from the Court, especially in front of a jury. I would obviously be overruled and would look bad to the jury. A sample of Judge Allen's questions are quite telling of the Judge's state of mind:

"Mr. Ahearn, that Friday, Saturday and Sunday had you noticed any injury to your wife's face like she had been hit by something?"

"Tell me what it was, will you?"

"What injury?"

"She thought she had pulled a muscle in her neck?"

"Aside from that conversation, had you seen any injuries?

"About her face or neck?"

Judge Allen then, per his custom, asked if any jurors had any questions of Dennis. Among the jurors' questions was the following:

"Did Michelle ever take two pills the same day before?"

Dennis responded, "Not that I can remember."

Following Dennis' testimony, Judge Allen called a noon recess. As we left the courtroom for a brief lunch, I complemented Dennis for doing a great job.

"I came close to breaking down," he said.

"Michelle, I expect you to do just as well, and I know you will," I said to her.

MICHELLE AHEARN

As we returned to the courtroom for the afternoon proceedings, Judge Allen took the bench asking me to proceed with my next witness.

"Your Honor, our next witness will be the Plaintiff, Michelle Ahearn."

Michelle took my arm and I escorted her to the witness stand. From the very first question Michelle's nervousness dissipated, and her vivacious personality became immediately apparent to the jury. She was succinct yet emotionally moving with her answers. She was an amazing witness, demonstrating tremendous courage in facing her situation and the trial itself. The jurors were obviously impressed with her. They hung on every word of her story as she laid it out from her early life, through the catastrophic illness that almost took her life, to living as a blind mother and wife.

I asked Michelle to describe to the jury the loss of everyday pleasures in her life. She choked up as she thought of how to answer that question, and just sat there for a minute trying to collect herself. Judge Allen then rudely said, "Mrs. Ahearn, would you please answer the question?" I was shocked that the Judge would be so rude to a noticeably distraught witness. As I scanned jurors' faces, it was obvious to me they did not appreciate what the judge did at that moment.

Michelle became very scared at the judge's comment answering softly:

"I don't enjoy anything as much as I used to . . . no matter what I do, I no longer enjoy it like I used to . . . I am blind . . . I do things to be doing them . . . I live with new fears, being alone in the house or in a crowd, answering the doorbell, receiving burns in attempts at cooking and ironing."

"Can you give the jury an example of some of the frustrations you face daily as a blind mother of three children?" I asked.

"I had a two-year-old I had to deal with taking care of. I was very worried where he was all the time. Could he get out the door of our home and into the street without me knowing it? The first thing I had to think about was how do I know where that child is? I finally came up with a solution. I tied little silver bells from Christmas packages to his shoes so that I could hear him as he moved around the house."

Then, lightening up her testimony, she said, "I was attempting to cook again for my family. I made a big pot of Italian minestrone soup for dinner. Dennis served the soup for me. The boys suddenly said, 'What's yellow and hard that is in the soup?' I replied that I didn't put anything like that into the soup. Dennis then said it looked like popcorn. I pulled out the plastic bag from the cupboard that I had used assuming it was a bag of Barley. Dennis said it was popcorn. It had been next to the bag of barley."

The jury laughed at her humor inserted into the story, but the jury was at the same time moved with emotion at the hardships she had to face as a blind mother raising three children. At times during her testimony, her emotions were close to the surface and she was struggling to avoid breaking down clearly to avoid invoking sympathy.

"Michelle, have you sought any professional help in dealing with your blindness?"

"I sought help from a psychiatrist. Although he told me he'd never treated a blind person before, he treated me for about a month and then left on a vacation to the Oregon Caves. When he returned and saw me for a routine visit, he commented to me, 'I never knew what it was like to be totally in the dark. When one closes their eyes, they still see light, but this was a total absence of light. I know how it feels to be completely confining. Michelle, you've been screwed!' I replied to him, "You know, Doc, tell me something I don't know."

There was no question in my mind the jury loved her and admired her courage in dealing with her blindness for the rest of her life. Marion's cross-examination of Michelle was brief and civil as would be expected. A harsh cross-examination on Michelle would certainly have been resented by the jury and backfired on the Defense.

Judge Allen then proceeded with what amounted to, in my view, a rude cross-examination of Michelle which again indicated bias. I could not object to the Judge's questions in front of the jury.

Judge Allen: "Did you see any literature on the subject of the 'Pill' that your sister had? Did you see any?"

Michelle had already answered this question from Marion which was clearly, "No." So there was no need for further repeating of the question by the Court.

The jurors' questions were few and much more polite such as:

"Did you ever take two pills the same day before?" to which
Michelle responded, "No."

∞

As Michelle left the witness stand, we were elated with the
wonderful impression she left on the jury. I thought to myself what
a great witness to end our case in chief. As our last witness, the
jurors' observation of this young mother of three, telling her story of
now living a life of blindness and its consequences would, without
a doubt, leave an indelible memory in their minds for at least the
remainder of the trial. Relying upon the principle that people will
remember best what they have seen and heard, first and last, this
confirmed this was a perfect place to end the presentation of our
case.

However, before we chose to rest our case, Harold and I
requested the Court to allow us a recess to discuss the matter
among ourselves. We had to be certain that we had presented
sufficient evidence to carry our burden of proof, i.e., that Ortho-
Novum was a *substantial factor* in causing Michelle's blindness.
If we had not carried our burden of proof, upon a motion by the
Defense, the Court would have the authority to toss the case out of
court at the moment we announced we had rested our case. This is
one of the many legal hurdles, under California law, that serves as
a check and balance in preventing an unmeritorious case from ever
reaching a jury's determination.

∞

After a short discussion, Harold and I agreed that we had presented
sufficient evidence to meet our burden of proof. We were pleased at

how well all our witnesses had testified. We further agreed that the cross-examinations by the Defense did not weaken our witnesses' credibility in any way. So, we concluded it was a good time to rest, and let Johnson & Johnson proceed with the presentation of their Defense.

There was much more documentary evidence we needed to introduce, such as scientific studies, case reports, and Ortho internal documents, but this would have to wait until we had the opportunity of cross-examination of Defense witnesses.

I announced to the Court and jury, "Your Honor, the Plaintiffs rest their case."

The Judge noted it was midday, and at Marion's request, he recessed the trial until the next morning to allow the Defense time to organize the presentation of their witnesses.

As we left the courthouse, Michelle discussed her dislike of Judge Allen. "I don't like the man, nor how he talked to me and treated me. My emotions float close to the surface. I tried really hard not to break down on the stand and evoke sympathy. I am scared, I don't think I made a good witness. It was intimidating. The last thing I wanted to do was hurt the case."

I immediately replied, "Michele, you did good. The jury loved you. They did not like what the judge did to you. The case is still strong." She calmed down and began to joke with me that I was still her F. Lee Baily and we parted for the day.

At this point of the trial we were all pleased with the manner in which our case was presented, but knowing the unpredictability of jurors in any trial, we were still far from confident on how it would end.

That evening, I summarized my thoughts in a conversation with Laura. Nine highly qualified and specialized medical doctors testified for the Plaintiffs. Five of them, Drs. Altshuler, Bettman, Leissring, Van Meter, and Overton, expressed opinions that (1) the "Pill" *causes* clotting/thrombosis and/or a predisposition thereto, and (2) that the "Pill" was, itself, a *substantial factor* in causing Plaintiff's blindness. All considered infection as present. However, some attributed the strep as merely a partial cause in the chain, a triggering device to thrombosis. They considered strep as working in combination with the predisposition to thrombosis caused by the "Pill." Others considered strep as merely an insignificant secondary factor in her illness and not a primary cause of her blindness.

Two other highly qualified witnesses from the Food and Drug Administration, Dr. Ley, the past FDA Commissioner, and Dr. McCleery, the FDA specialist on warnings, testified that the "Pill" causes thrombosis, and further that the warnings from the pharmaceutical industry were inaccurate and misleading. Mr. Preston, a current employed detail man for Ortho admitted that physicians were never told of any causal relationship or risk between the "Pill" and thrombosis by Ortho's representatives when making sales calls. Lastly, Dr. Harris, a local practicing physician who was our first witness in the case, authenticated several letters between him and Dr. Cronk, the medical director for Ortho, confirming his direct experience with a triple challenge and response case of the "Pill" causing life threatening thrombosis to his wife. I thought we presented a strong case and Laura agreed.

As I began to look forward in anticipation of the Defense presentation of their witnesses, I knew I could rely upon a common courtesy in trial. We had alerted the Defense which witnesses we would be presenting a day in advance so that Marion would have an opportunity to prepare his cross-examination, and Marion agreed to do the same. Complying with that agreement, Marion advised us the first witness for the next morning would be Dr. Kosmin, Michelle's treating hematologist, followed by Dr. Lippe, her treating neurosurgeon. Normally, that would be a shock to us that treating doctors would cooperate with their own patient's adversary to defeat his patient's personal injury claim, but in this case we, of course, knew that was coming.

CHAPTER 9
JOHNSON & JOHNSON FIGHTS BACK

I awakened the next morning with my thoughts shifting to what we were facing next and the strategy we had adapted. The primary Defense theory would be that the "Pill" did not cause Michelle's blindness. Rather, Ortho contended the *infection alone* was the *sole* cause, and the "Pill" had nothing to do with her blindness. Further, Ortho contended there was inadequate evidence the "Pill" caused blood clotting/thrombosis disorders in *any* woman, nor was there a risk of such since thrombosis occurs spontaneously in the population.

We knew they would rely heavily upon the testimony of three of the six doctors who treated Michelle during her hospitalization for this illness, each of whom had cooperated fully with Ortho. This factor raised a major concern in our minds knowing that jurors have a tendency to accept the opinions of treating physicians over that of retained experts—"hired guns."

These doctors knew of Harold's extensive past experience as a treating physician. I thought our chance of getting truthful medical answers from the treating doctors would be increased if Harold did the cross-examination rather than me. I was the one who had previously contacted these doctors to solicit their help in testifying for Michelle. At that time, they showed extreme resentment toward me for having filed a lawsuit alleging that Ortho-Novum caused her blindness. They were each personally convinced I was wrong in blaming Michelle's blindness on the Ortho-Novum and looked upon the case as a threat to all physicians prescribing the "Pill."

In any event, I was the enemy in their eyes, and I didn't feel too kindly about them either. So, I felt it would be wiser if someone other than me did the cross-examination. A treating doctor on treating doctors was our adopted strategy. I also thought since I had done all the direct examination in our case presentation, it would be wise for the jury to experience Harold in action.

A tall, slender, good-looking man in his early fifties, Harold spoke in a low tenor voice which he could use in an authoritative and commanding manner, yet always respectful and civil. He would use short, but articulate sentences that would leave little room for a hostile medical witness to evade. All of this, when added to a natural command of medical terminology and an extensive knowledge in human physiology, would contribute to Harold being ideal as a cross-examiner of these three hostile treating physicians we had to face.

MARTIN KOSMIN, M.D.

The next morning Harold and I made our way to Judge Allen's courtroom feeling confident the trial was going as well as could be expected, if not better. Harold and I worked together the previous evening preparing him for his cross-examination of Dr. Kosmin and the others. We knew from the medical records what Dr. Kosmin would ultimately be compelled to admit when confronted with his own medical entries and we were comfortable with that. Harold and I had discussed how Dr. Kosmin's own medical notes in the hospital records acknowledged thrombosis was at work in Michelle when he first saw her, and the notes clearly indicated he did not know why.

As we took our positions at counsel table that morning ready to proceed, we were hit with another surprise. As Judge Allen took the bench, he asked counsel to approach. He told us the clerk had received a call from a juror who had a family emergency and would not be able to attend the rest of the trial. We all agreed to use our second alternate juror to replace her. The jury at this point now consisted of nine women and three men, plus a male alternate.

∽

We returned to counsel table and Judge Allen asked Marion to call his witness to the stand.

"Your Honor, the Defense will call Dr. Martin Kosmin to the witness stand as our first witness."

Marion started the usual questioning to establish the witness' credentials as a qualified physician with a specialty in hematology (a blood specialist). He had Dr. Kosmin describe how he had been called in to see Michelle by Dr. Lippe, her neurosurgeon. Dr. Kosmin contended Dr. Lippe brought him into the case because he thought there was a problem of infection in the blood. Dr. Kosmin who happened to arrive at her bedside before Dr. Lippe, was the first to see her when she entered emergency.

As I listened to this testimony, I thought to myself, if Dr. Lippe really believed the problem was an infection in the blood, why didn't he call in an infectious disease expert, rather than a hematologist? A hematologist would be the logical referral if Dr. Lippe was thinking thrombosis might be the problem.

Dr. Kosmin testified he took over as the primary treating physician. He described how he first examined Michelle while in emergency around 8 p.m. and immediately admitted her to the hospital with a provisional diagnosis of "facial cellulitis," an infection in swollen facial tissue on the left side of her face and eye. In response to appropriate questioning by Marion, he detailed his treatment and involvement during the entire course of her hospitalization, emphasizing the strep infection that had been found in her blood stream. He strongly denied any possible causal role of thrombosis and the oral contraceptive in Michelle's illness.

∾

Harold initiated his cross-examination of Dr. Kosmin by probing into his background and experience. He established that although Dr. Kosmin was assigned as the primary treating doctor for Michelle, his testimony revealed he was the least experienced physician than any doctor who had testified so far. Although a board-certified internist and hematologist, he had been in private practice for only one and a half years beyond fellowship and residency training at the time he treated Michelle, and only five years total before leaving the practice of medicine.

The last two and a half years, prior to this Court testimony, he reluctantly admitted he had been occupied as a medical consultant to the legal department of a major pharmaceutical manufacturer,

Merck, Sharp & Dohme Research Labs. His primary job was as a consultant on drug product liability cases defending his employer. Wouldn't his work background create some bias in Ortho's favor? The weaknesses in his testimony that surfaced during his direct examination were exploited by the calm civil demeanor and direct questioning style of Harold's excellent cross-examination.

As cross-examination continued, Dr. Kosmin revealed that although orbital cellulitis was his initial diagnosis of Michelle's illness, he admitted that hers was the only case he had ever seen. "I have never seen a case anything like this," in terms of swelling and permanent blindness. He conceded the thought that Michelle might go blind never even entered his mind when he first saw her. A little shamelessly, he admitted to Harold "It was not until the next day, the 17th, that I realized she could be fatally ill." He also admitted he found her "jugular vein *thrombosed*," but conceded he did not know what areas of the head it drained. As I heard this concession of thrombosis, I saw the turning point in his testimony.

Harold then pointed out in questioning, ". . . wouldn't it be the ophthalmic and cavernous sinus area of the head that it drains?" Dr. Kosmin repeated he didn't know. He embarrassingly admitted he did not have the "faintest idea" as to the location of the pterygoid plexus, and most significantly that he did not know if the "Pill" caused clotting. Like all the other treating doctors, he admitted he never even asked Michelle if she was on the "Pill." He confirmed that the entire hospital record failed to show a single notation by any doctor, nurse, or other person, that Michelle had been taking the "Pill." This medical fact, obviously, was never even a consideration in the minds nor medical diagnosis by anyone during her entire hospitalization.

As cross-examination continued, the weaknesses in Dr. Kosmin's testimony became glaring, especially his lack of knowledge and memory of specifics in her case. He traveled 3,000 miles from the East Coast to testify yet failed to review the hospital records containing his own notes. Nor did he research the medical literature on any of the medical issues in the case, despite such activity constituting his current job as a consultant to the legal department in similar product liability cases.

When asked to explain his current job, he responded, "It is too complicated to explain. I am not sure I understand it myself." His testimony revealed serious flaws in his competency, credibility, and his ability to perceive, retain, and recall significant information in this once-in-a-lifetime case. The ordinary person, let alone a physician, certainly should be able to recall such a unique case, indelibly recorded in the mind as a result of such an unusual experience.

"Doctor, did you personally withdraw the blood samples for culture?" Harold asked.

"I have no recollection."

"Did you take a throat culture?"

"I can't recall."

"Do you know when it was taken?"

"I can't recall."

"Doctor, were you aware of the fact that Michelle did not have any fever up to the time she entered the hospital?"

"I don't know."

"Doctor, did you believe the infection started in the orbit of the swollen eye?"

"I don't know."

"Doctor, why did you write down your initial diagnosis as "*orbital cellulitis?*"

"It may have been that I just thought that was the most significant thing to write down at the time." Dr. Kosmin contended.

At the time of Michelle's admission to the hospital, he did not know where the infection started and testified at the time of trial that he still did not know. The location of the initial infection in the throat was the primary basis for the Defense theory that a strep throat was the *sole* cause of Michelle's blindness, yet this primary treating physician presented by the Defense "did not know!" Despite his initial diagnosis of orbital cellulitis, when Harold asked, "Doctor, what is the first symptom of *orbital cellulitis?*"

Dr. Kosmin cavalierly replied, "I haven't the faintest idea."

Dr. Kosmin did not notice Michelle's left eye bulging on admission, but admitted it was at some time later. When asked if he had seen any purulent secretions coming out of that eye, he again replied, "I don't know." The lack of any hard evidence of infection being observed by Dr. Kosmin, particularly in the swollen orbit of the eye and face, created doubt as to his diagnosis of orbital or facial infectious cellulitis, as distinguished from swelling caused by pressure from thrombosis.

When Harold asked, "Could you tell us where you think the streptococcus made its way into the bloodstream?"

Dr. Kosmin again replied, "I haven't the faintest idea."

He conceded that there was no doubt in his mind that phlebitis or thrombophlebitis can occur without infection.

Dr. Kosmin agreed that spinal fluid pressure of 440, as found in Michelle, was "a very severe elevated pressure, and that severe headache is one symptom of increased intra-cranial pressure that worsens as the pressure builds up." This concurred with Dr. Overton's explanation (Plaintiff's expert neurosurgeon). Dr. Kosmin further corroborated Dr. Overton's explanation that "increased intra-cranial pressure may be due to obstruction of the veins that drain the blood out of the head." When asked if this could result in blood cells appearing in the spinal fluid, he acknowledged, "I really don't know." When asked if he considered that the 920 white blood cell count in Michelle's spinal fluid might be the result of intra-cranial pressure, he replied, "I don't know whether I considered it or not."

The tragic surprise that awaited the treating doctors is nowhere better illustrated than by Dr. Kosmin's following testimony:

"Doctor, you didn't realize when you first saw her that you were dealing with something which might cause her to go blind within the next couple of days, did you?"

"No, that was not something that even entered my mind . . ."

When he described a palpable cord in Michelle's neck, he was asked if he thought it might have been a thrombosed or clotted vein. He replied, "I think that's what I thought." Anticoagulant medication, such as Heparin, was generally used at the time to dissolve blood clots and treat thrombosis.

Harold asked, "Doctor, why was it that Heparin was not started until about *13 hours after you* and Dr. Lippe discussed giving Michelle anticoagulants?"

He again cavalierly replied, "I have no idea."

He conceded that he was concerned about the clotting potential in Michelle from the beginning and that is why he eventually gave her Heparin. The hospital records indicated that initially he requested the hospital to obtain a different and more powerful anti-coagulant, Urokinase, but it was not available.

Here again, the cross-examination testimony of Dr. Kosmin strongly supported substantial thrombosis as the mechanism of Michelle's blindness, and not a strep infection alone. Yet he testified on direct examination that he did not think clotting had *anything* to do with Michelle's blindness.

As to the sequence of important bacteriological events, he had no knowledge:

"Well, do you think the bacteria in the bloodstream preceded the cellulitis or followed it?" Harold asked.

"I have no idea."

"Is it your testimony that you think it was a cellulitis or a bloodstream infection or both that caused the headache starting on Saturday night, the 15th of February?"

"No, I think I don't know what caused her headache . . ."

When asked where the infection originated, he said, "I don't know where it started."

The absence of support in the medical literature, or otherwise, for the defense position on causation was sharply put in focus by Dr. Kosmin when Harold asked, "Have you ever heard of any other case or read about any other case of total bilateral blindness resulting from a streptococcal infection?"

"I can't say that I have," Dr. Kosmin confirmed.

As to the reason for Michelle's blindness, Dr. Kosmin summarized his own view and understanding of the views of his fellow treating doctors when he said, ". . . we did not come up with any good explanation." When asked if he was aware that the entire hospital record failed to show a single notation that Michelle had been taking the "Pill," Dr. Kosmin curtly replied, "If you tell me that, I believe it."

Whether or not the "Pill" contributed to Michelle's blindness was, of course, the most important medical issue in this case. Dr. Kosmin's contribution to resolving this issue followed:

"Doctor, do you have an opinion as to whether or not the birth control pill in this case had anything to do with contributing to Michelle's blindness?"

"Whether it had anything to do?"

"Yes." Harold said.

"In any manner, shape or form?" Dr. Kosmin asked.

"Yes."

"I have no idea." Dr. Kosmin finally responded.

⟨⟩

As I listened to Dr. Kosmin's testimony, my worries about the damage these treating doctors might do to our case substantially evaporated. He gave us the truth we needed, i.e., massive thrombosis occurred in Michelle during this dreadful illness. That put the strep infection in a secondary place in the potential list of causal factors causing her blindness. Further, the fact that this treating doctor could not identify a single source of the strep infection found only in Michelle's blood, should have eliminated strep as the *sole* cause of Michelle's blindness.

The delay of thirteen hours from when thrombosis was found before treatment with an anti-coagulant was certain to raise questions in the jury's mind. In fact, that same question had arisen in a juror's mind during Dr. Bettman's testimony earlier, when she asked:

"If Michelle had been prescribed the Heparin on her admission to the hospital, what are the chances that her blindness might have been prevented?"

Dr. Bettman explained that not having personally seen her, he couldn't say with any certainty. However, Dr. Kosmin, as a hematologist, had seen Michelle during her entire hospitalization so he had no excuse for not recognizing that any delay in anti-coagulation treatment was crucial in preventing Michelle's blindness.

There was little redirect examination by Marion, and it was of no real significance. Dr. Kosmin was excused by the Court and I sighed in relief. If the jury had been carefully listening to his testimony, they would come to realize this treating physician ultimately provided support to our contention that thrombosis, and not strep, was the major cause at play in Michelle. Now my concern was whether the remaining two treating physicians yet to testify, would somehow undermine this testimony of Dr. Kosmin.

After excusing Dr. Kosmin, the Court called a recess. I approached Michelle and Dennis and asked for their impression of Dr. Kosmin's testimony.

Michelle replied, "It infuriated me, even though I had thanked him for coming to testify for me when we met in the hallway before he took the stand—I forgot he was there to testify for the Defense. I knew he was going to work for a drug company, but didn't know in what capacity. I felt this man's testimony, as an educated man, never mind a doctor, demonstrated he purposely didn't review any records, or refresh his memory, so he wouldn't know anything. I was his patient, but because of his employment by a drug company,

I felt he was intimidated by the drug company to not do anything to help my cause."

PHILLIP LIPPE, M.D.

We returned to the courtroom after the break and Marion announced, "Your Honor, the Defense calls Dr. Phillip Lippe to the stand."

Dr. Phillip Lippe had only been practicing neurosurgery for a short time, yet by the time he testified he was already quite well known and respected by the medical community in San Jose. Typical of some neurosurgeons, he displayed an air of arrogance and certainty despite being somewhat young for a neurosurgeon. Brain surgeons were looked up to with unusual awe and respect, not only by the general public, but also by the medical world.

As the treating neurosurgeon called in by Dr. Gossack to see Michelle in the hospital at the time of her admission, he had the advantage of speaking with Dr. Gossack on the history of Michelle's initial signs and symptoms. He received the call because he just happened to be at the hospital already making hospital rounds that Sunday evening. Due to the extreme inexplicable migraine-type headache Michelle was experiencing at the time, Dr. Gossack felt a neurological complication may have been involved, and he certainly had confidence in the competency of Dr. Lippe.

Marion started his direct examination in the usual way by having Dr. Lippe testify to his educational background and qualifications, which were impressive. Dr. Lippe testified that he was board-certified in neurosurgery and had been in practice within his specialty for about four years when he saw Michelle in emergency that evening. After he examined her, he explained that he turned her primary care over to Dr. Kosmin and did not see Michelle again for over twelve hours, and only intermittently thereafter.

Marion had him review for the jury the entries in the hospital medical chart of each involvement he had with Michelle during her hospitalization. Most surprisingly to us during the course of his testimony, the doctor did not take a strong position that strep caused her blindness. The entire direct examination appeared almost insignificant to the Defense's contentions, other than demonstrating that Dr. Lippe had a complete lack of opinion as to why Michelle was blind. "I have no further questions at this time, your Honor," Marion stated.

Harold rose from counsel table.

"Good morning, Dr. Lippe. At the time, you were treating Michelle in the hospital you did not conclude that strep caused her blindness, is that accurate?"

"That's true, I am not certain why Michelle was blind . . . I really cannot tell you exactly why she is blind."

Then came the biggest surprise in my mind.

"Would you agree that thrombosis was a significant factor in Michelle's illness?"

"There was no doubt in my mind that thrombosis *did* play a part in Michelle's illness, including extensive thrombosis over the facial and jugular veins and some degree of obstruction of the cavernous sinus," he admitted.

He postulated that Michelle's blindness was due to a "mechanical pressure related phenomenon" and not due exclusively to cellulitis or soft tissue inflammation. He conceded it was due to a sequence of events including a "thrombotic process," a unique chain of events never seen before by him.

The foregoing testimony was not only contrary to the Defense contentions of strep alone as the cause, but amazingly strongly supported our experts' contentions that thrombosis was the *major* cause in the chain of events.

There were, however, a few discrepancies in his testimony that further strengthened our case. On direct examination, he had claimed that bilateral blindness from orbital cellulitis, was well recognized in medicine, contrary to the testimony of every other expert at trial from both sides.

However, when challenged by Harold on cross-examination the following colloquy occurred:

"Well, Doctor, where is it well recognized that *bilateral* total blindness may occur from orbital cellulitis? Is it written up somewhere?"

"I'm sure it is."

"Can you tell us where?"

"I cannot, sir."

"But you did find it?"

"Yes."

"Well did you make a notation or make a copy of an article or . . ."

"Why should I?"

Harold followed this response from Dr. Lippe by getting him to admit he required me to pay him, as her treating doctor, an hourly fee for consultation time on Michelle's case, and, thereafter, consulted for three to five hours with three lawyers representing Johnson & Johnson on this case, with neither Michelle's nor my consent. At the Defense's request, he further reviewed deposition transcripts of other expert physicians in this case and then consulted with another Defense expert witness. All of this work was done in preparation for Dr. Lippe to testify as an expert on behalf of the Defense.

Dr. Lippe continued to demonstrate further weaknesses in his testimony admitting that he had only a "vague idea" of the location of the pterygoid plexus (in the cheek area of the face) and had "never heard of thrombophlebitis of the pterygoid plexus." Further, he "would not recognize it if it occurred." Thrombophlebitis of the pterygoid plexus was confirmed in Michelle by several other experts who testified at trial, both Defense and Plaintiff.

When another treating physician, Dr. Finkel, an ophthalmologist, noted the inability of Michelle to see any light whatsoever, Dr. Lippe admitted he recorded in Michelle's medical chart that this was a "common complication of cavernous sinus thrombosis." He further conceded in his testimony that cavernous sinus thrombosis as seen "these days" is secondary to some process *other* than infection. As I heard this opinion, I thought for a moment he must be our witness. This statement by Dr. Lippe clearly tended to exclude infection as the sole cause of Michelle's blindness.

Dr. Lippe testified that he had no opinion as to when the septicemia started, but admitted "classically it is associated with shaking, fevers and chills." Michelle never had these before entering the hospital.

Another major gain for our position occurred when Dr. Lippe agreed with Harold that Michelle's severe headache was not from a strep throat or septicemia and admitted she "did not have a sore throat when seen in emergency."

When Harold asked, "Doctor, did a strep throat ever exist in Michelle?"

Dr. Lippe confessed, "We certainly never proved that point."

Dr. Lippe admitted he never looked at Dr. Gossack's records on Michelle (as distinguished from the hospital records). He therefore had no knowledge of her medical history for this illness during the thirty hours before his own examination, other than the severe migraine headache communicated to him by Dr. Gossack. He, like all the other hospital treating physicians, conceded he did not ask, nor did he know, that Michelle was on the "Pill" at that time. Of course, no one, from the moment of her admission to the hospital, ever asked her that vital question. Was the failure to ask a result of pharmaceutical manufacturers' failure to warn physicians of serious thrombosis risks from the "Pill?"

A total unexpected bonus came from Dr. Lippe near the end of Harold's cross-examination:

"Do you have an opinion at this time as to whether the 'Pill' could cause blood clotting in some women?"

"*Now*, I believe the 'Pill' *probably causes abnormal clotting* in some women."

If only he had that belief when he saw Michelle in 1969. Would he have asked her or Dr. Gossack, if she was on the "Pill?" And if he had, would he and Dr. Kosmin have started anticoagulants much sooner? Would that have stopped or even dissolved the thrombosis before the blood flow to the optic nerves became blocked? In short, would that have then saved Michelle's sight? Several jurors had asked expert witnesses this very question to which each witness evaded a conclusive answer.

Taking a further perspective, what if Ortho had not successfully blocked the recommendation of the FDA OB-GYN Advisory Committee to change the warning to a "cause and effect" relationship between the "Pill" and abnormal blood clotting back in late 1968. Would it have been more likely, in that event, that both Dr. Lippe and/or Dr. Kosmin would have been aware of the potential of the "Pill" causing clotting, at that earlier time? They again might have asked Michelle or Dr. Gossack if she was on the "Pill," and consequently administer anticoagulants much more timely, thereby saving her vision. Obviously, Dr. Lippe would have been receptive to such a warning in that he was open to such causation in 1974, at the time of this trial. If these circumstances were true, doesn't this make Ortho and Johnson & Johnson the true culprits?

Marion could do nothing to rehabilitate Dr. Lippe's testimony on redirect.

There was still one more surprise to come. Judge Allen then asked Dr. Lippe a question concerning past testimony of Dr. Overton, our neurosurgeon expert witness. In response, Dr. Lippe, not only differed with the opinions of Dr. Overton, but openly criticized his competency and integrity. I immediately thought what a foolish mistake to make in a jury trial. Dr. Overton seemed to be well accepted by the jury who themselves had asked him many questions. As a trial lawyer, I knew for one expert witness to attack the competency and integrity of another expert witness, never goes well with a jury.

Judge Allen then allowed questions for Dr. Lippe from some jurors.

One juror asked, "Do you have an opinion whether Michelle had a cavernous sinus thrombosis?"

He made the major concession, in his response, that Michelle *may* have had a "cavernous sinus thrombosis." He conceded that septicemia occurring secondary to swelling could not be ruled out. In other words, the process of swelling itself, caused by thrombosis alone, could have allowed a strep infection to get into the blood stream secondarily.

Marion asked that Dr. Lippe be excused as a witness and the Court adjourned for the day.

Contrary to our expectations, Dr. Lippe's testimony, particularly on cross-examination, did not help the Defense at all but certainly helped our case. As I heard his testimony, I wondered why he refused to work with us on behalf of his patient, but rather chose to cooperate with the Defense. He achieved the opposite, fortunately for us.

Marion advised us that among the witnesses he would be calling the next day was Dr. Sogg. We were now down to the last treating doctor the Defense would be calling to the stand. Harold and I left the courtroom feeling comfortable that a potentially bad day turned out to be not so bad, after all.

As we left the courtroom, I asked Michelle her thoughts on Dr. Lippe.

She angrily answered, "He wasn't so nice. To me, he came across very cold and uncaring. It was like you're a piece of meat. No human feeling in there." Dennis agreed. We parted and Harold and I returned to my office to work on cross-examination of Dr. Sogg and the other Defense witnesses.

RICHARD SOGG, M.D.

We arrived at the courthouse a half-hour early to deal evidentiary issues the Judge wanted to discuss before the jury was brought in. After our discussions, we waited for the jury to arrive, and my thoughts drifted to my first meeting with Dr. Sogg. I was, at first, somewhat impressed with his apparent knowledge and acclaimed expertise. I noted his Harvard degree on his wall. I remember him as being quite articulate in conversation, and, unlike either Dr. Kosmin or Dr. Lippe, he seemed to have a genuine interest in understanding my reasons for believing the "Pill" caused Michele's blindness. For these reasons, I did not hesitate in sharing with him substantial evidence we had accumulated to support Michelle's case. I was assuming he would be testifying on our behalf as her treating neuro-ophthalmologist which could be powerful in the jury's eyes.

Although he was charging me $100.00 an hour for our meeting in which I was sharing with him the evidence of our case, I was led to believe I was truly educating him on the abundance of medical research on oral contraceptives he would not know existed as a neuro-ophthalmologist. He appeared not to be aware of the many adverse reaction reports on eye complications from the "Pill," nor the existence of the challenge and response cases. I even shared with him the triple challenge and response case of Dr. Harris who also practiced in Santa Clara County. I did not expect him to be aware of this medical literature at that time period (early 1970's).

Trusting him as my client's treating physician, I shared confidential information such as the opinions of Dr. Bettman on the case.

In early 1974, when his deposition was taken by the Defense, I realized I had made a huge mistake in trusting his intentions in the case. His opinion expressed in deposition was that the sole cause of Michele's blindness was the "*strep infection.*" He contended that the "portal of entry" for the strep was her "cut finger" she experienced one to two weeks before hospitalization. He testified in that deposition that the strep thereby entered her blood stream eventually causing facial and orbital cellulitis that, itself, created pressure that cut off blood flow to her optic nerves. I surmised from the research he disclosed at the deposition that he must have joined the Defense camp and was compensated for his time as their expert. Suspicion and apprehension began to set in as it appeared he had been communicating the information I provided him to the Defense. Knowing all this, I became concerned that because he was a treating doctor, as well as a hired expert for the Defense, the jury might find him credible and buy his "cut finger" theory.

The past experiences with all three treating physicians, Drs. Kosmin, Lippe, and Sogg caused me to develop a substantial dislike for all three, but especially Dr. Sogg. Why would treating physicians be so willing to work against their own patients' interest in such major litigation? They were not the ones being sued. With such bitterness toward them, I realized again I had made the right decision in choosing Harold to do their cross-examination. I was too emotionally angered with each of them.

Harold, as a past treating doctor, was not so offended by what they had done.

All three were competent physicians dedicated to the practice of medicine but trusting of Johnson & Johnson. Their first opportunity to use a stethoscope as young medical students in medical school was most probably because it was made available by Johnson & Johnson. Pharmaceutical companies, and especially Johnson & Johnson, provided medical equipment free of charge to the major medical schools throughout the United States as part of their promotional activities. After all, this was no ordinary corporation. They were like motherhood and apple pie to the general American public, and more so to medical students and physicians. Johnson & Johnson had been around for over a century and made products safely used over many decades such as band-aids and baby powder. Certainly, they could be trusted and relied upon not to have produced a drug that would cause severe harm.

So, when Ortho's personnel visited these three treating doctors and told them that their product, "Ortho-Novum" was safe, as believed by most practicing physicians at that time, they also believed them, contrary to what any patient's lawyer, like myself, might contend. Not just the entire medical world, but also the general population believed the "Pill" was safe, and a great gift to society. They would conclude from all this experience that any contrary claims were the sole result of greedy trial lawyers out to get rich filing unmeritorious lawsuits.

By cooperating with Johnson & Johnson, they believed they were upholding sound science and good medical practice. It therefore became easy for them to become convinced that Michelle's blindness had to be the sole result of an infection, and certainly not from the oral contraceptive distributed by such a good standing corporation. Of course, these practicing physicians had never seen all the hard, negative evidence we had obtained through the powerful legal process of discovery.

The night before, we discussed how Dr. Sogg's credentials would be impossible to impeach, and that our approach had to be to dismantle the unmeritorious basis for the opinions expressed in his deposition.

The next morning, I noticed the volume of spectators was diminishing as the trial slumbered on. Judge Allen took the bench, the jury returned to their assigned seats, and Judge Allen instructed Marion, "You may proceed with your next witness."

"Thank you, your Honor, we would like to call Dr. Sogg to the witness stand."

Marion started out in the usual format having Dr. Sogg provide the jury with his educational background and experience. Dr. Sogg testified that he was a board-certified ophthalmologist since 1962 and currently teaching ophthalmology and neuro-ophthalmology two days a week at Stanford University Medical School. He noted that he was on the faculty there with Dr. Bettman.

He explained to the jury how he was called in to consult on the evening of February 19th, three days after Michelle's hospitalization and the day Dr. Finkel discovered she was blind. I listened hoping the jury would remember Michelle was no longer in acute distress at that time, but was recovering having received massive doses of antibiotics and anti-coagulation medication.

As I anticipated, he emphatically expressed his expert opinion as to the mechanism of blindness:

"The cut finger became the portal of entry for the strep infection . . . the strep then spread into her blood stream . . . eventually

landing in the orbit of the eye, her face, and pharynx [throat area] .
. . causing cellulitis . . . extreme inflammation in those areas."

He stated the "cellulitis became the mechanism that caused
her blindness . . . swelling that caused the backup of blood supply
to the optic nerves." As I listened, I observed Dr. Sogg becoming
somewhat uncomfortable while testifying. I wondered what the
jury thought of his opinion of causation having heard other expert
witnesses, both Plaintiff and Defense, testify that the "cut finger"
was irrelevant to the case since it occurred two weeks before her
illness.

Dr. Sogg backed up his theory of causation by claiming
Michelle had a "history of tonsillitis, recurrent chills, sweating
episodes, and shivering spells." When I heard this, I knew he was
over-reaching and hoped the jury realized the same. He obviously
never reviewed Dr. Gossack's records which clearly dispelled that
history. Further, this testimony contradicted the lay testimony of
Michelle, her friend Alice, and Dennis as well, verifying factually,
no prior existence of any of those symptoms until she had entered
the hospital.

Dr. Sogg concluded his direct testimony with his opinion that
". . . strep infection was the sole cause of Michelle's blindness and
the Ortho-Novum had nothing to do with it."

Marion announced to the Court, "No further questions, your
Honor."

Harold then began his well-prepared cross-examination.

"Good afternoon Dr. Sogg. We have previously met?"

"Yes."

"Doctor, in the diagnostic testing you performed on Michelle,
you observed engorgement of the veins which drain the optic

nerves, ribbons of veins distended with blood clotting, is that correct?"

"Yes."

"You further observed in Michelle an elevated retina in her eyes which to you indicted a backup of blood draining from the retina. True?"

"Yes, Sir."

"According to your entry in Michelle's hospital chart, you further observed a lack of venous pulsation in both eyes indicating to you an obstruction to blood flowing out of the veins. Correct?"

"Correct."

"Then, isn't it true, Doctor, that no doubt existed in your mind that venous obstruction was a substantial factor in the overall problem that resulted in Michelle's blindness?"

"Absolutely." Dr. Sogg confirmed.

This testimony, of course, strongly corroborating a thrombotic event as a substantial cause of Michelle's blindness, undercut his prior direct testimony that a strep infection was the sole cause.

Harold then directed Dr. Sogg to his diagnosis in the hospital medical chart: "bilateral retro bulbar neuritis with disc edema" (inflammation of the optic nerves and swelling of the optic disc).

"Doctor, in your entry in the hospital chart you ascribed the three etiologies to explain your diagnosis: 1) passive edema which is swelling of the nerve due to increased pressure in the brain; 2) direct invasion of the optic nerve by streptococcus organisms, and 3) clotting of the vessels which nourish the optic nerve. As to your second etiology of strep invasion directly into the optic nerve, can you show me in the records where a single organism of streptococcus was ever found in Michelle's eyes, orbits, face, head, throat, or anywhere in her entire body other than her blood stream?"

"No," he embarrassingly acknowledged.

"Doctor, have you ever heard of such a case?"

"No," he again more quietly responded.

"Dr. Sogg, wouldn't fever and chills be the *initial symptoms* of a streptococcal septicemia [infection in the blood stream]?

"Yes," he said strongly.

"And that the early symptoms to be expected with orbital cellulitis would be pain, redness, swelling and tenderness in and about the eye, as well as severe fever?" Harold asked.

"Yes, and she had those," he said, completely unaware that Dr. Gossack, who first saw her with complaints of severe headache, had examined her for such symptoms and found none.

Harold continued, "Doctor, you agreed with Dr. Kosmin seeking a clot-dissolving enzyme, Urokinase, to treat Michelle for thrombosis, a fast working anticoagulant used in emergency situations, true?"

"Yes."

"Very unfortunately, it was not available in the hospital to you physicians at that time?"

"Yes, so we ordered Heparin."

I reflected on this great testimony unfolding in front of our eyes. If both treating physicians were seeking a powerful anticoagulant, wouldn't it appear to the jury these physicians well knew they were dealing with a major clotting situation? Wouldn't this very conduct corroborate the existence of a clotting mechanism, rather than infection, as being the most probable scenario in their minds at this crucial time of treatment? I hoped this would register in the jurors' minds as well.

Dr. Sogg admitted that he knew from a venogram, which is the study of blood flow through the veins, taken seventeen days after Michelle's onset of illness, that it demonstrated occluded (clotted) veins. In my mind at that time, and hopefully the jury's, the only question that could remain in any treating physician's mind is "what made her clot?" These treating physicians knew she had a strep infection from a blood culture despite finding no origin of such, but they did not know at that time the most crucial fact, i.e. that she had been on the "Pill." They never asked.

Harold's examination continued, "Dr. Sogg, do you admit that it is difficult for a physician to distinguish the diagnosis of orbital cellulitis from a cavernous sinus thrombosis?"

"Yes."

"You knew that Michelle's ophthalmologist, Dr. Finkle, who examined her vision on February 17th, reached a clinical assessment at that time that Michelle presented a full picture of cavernous sinus thrombosis?"

"I agree with him."

With this admission, Dr. Sogg and Dr. Finkle, the two treating ophthalmologists, provided further corroborating evidence that the mechanism of thrombosis was a substantial contributor to Michelle's blindness. Thus, on cross-examination, both treating ophthalmologists supported the same mechanism of blindness as testified to by Plaintiffs' experts as well, i.e. *a cavernous sinus thrombosis.*

Dr. Sogg's original testimony on direct examination by Ortho, that infection alone from her blood stream caused her blindness, through the mechanism of cellulitis, subsequently fell apart in this cross-examination. He was further impeached by the testimony of the primary treating doctor, Dr. Kosmin, the hematologist, that none of the treating doctors (including Dr. Sogg) understood what caused her blindness. Dr. Sogg in his direct testimony had blamed the cut finger, two weeks prior to the onset of illness, as the source of the strep infection which then floated around in her blood stream all that time, eventually landing in the orbit, face, and pharynx. Dr. Lippe, the Defense neurosurgeon, had previously testified that the cut finger was irrelevant to her illness.

Dr. Sogg specifically conceded to several critical, factual issues within his testimony such as: 1) no infected lymph nodes were palpable in Michelle's neck, 2) that an obstruction existed of the venous return from the cavernous sinus which can lead to swelling and redness of mucous membrane of the nose, throat, eye, orbit and face, rather than from infection, i.e., those symptoms that later appeared during Michelle's hospitalization, 3) that thrombosis of the jugular vein can lead to swelling such as Michelle demonstrated at the beginning of her illness, 4) that Dr. Kosmin had palpated a thrombosed jugular vein on Michelle, and 5) that thrombophlebitis can lead to inflammation of veins and surrounding tissue, *without infection*. All of the foregoing corroborated the testimony of Plaintiffs' experts.

A final understanding of why Dr. Sogg initially limited his diagnosis of orbital cellulitis surfaced when the subject of the role of the "Pill" was addressed to him. He first learned that Michelle was on the "Pill" many months later when we told him during our meeting.

When asked by Harold during cross-examination, "Dr. Sogg, do oral contraceptives cause blood clotting in some women?"

He responded, "I don't know."

Harold then presented him with a hypothetical question: "What if the 'Pill' does create a predisposition toward thrombophlebitis and an infection is added to that predisposition, would you agree *that combination* would increase the risk that she would ultimately develop thrombosis?"

"An increased risk to thrombophlebitis would then exist," he admitted.

As seen earlier, this was the exact testimony of Plaintiffs' expert ophthalmologist, Dr. Bettman.

When Dr. Sogg was further asked, "Are you aware of any case ever reported in the medical literature where bilateral blindness ensued within three days after the onset of symptoms of either orbital cellulitis or cavernous sinus thrombosis?"

He responded, "No, Michelle's case was the most dramatic case of this kind I have ever seen. I performed a diligent search of the medical literature which did not disclose anything like it."

Thus, Dr. Sogg corroborated Plaintiffs' expert, Dr. Bettmen, on the key factual issue of causation—*an increased risk of thrombosis in one already predisposed by the "Pill."*

At one point in his testimony, Dr. Sogg severely overreached in his attempt to justify his original diagnosis of orbital cellulitis. In his direct examination by Ortho he contended that there were other similar cases reported in the medical literature of bilateral blindness from orbital cellulitis, including two cases in which the patients went "completely blind" from streptococcus cultured from their orbits. This was the same bacteria cultured from Michelle's blood while hospitalized.

On cross-examination Harold showed Dr. Sogg copies of these particular medical reports from the literature, and asked, "Dr. Sogg, do those reports which you cited refer to blindness in both eyes of those patients?"

"No, only one eye in each," Dr. Sogg embarrassingly admitted.

"And was evidence of the origin of strep infection found in the paranasal sinuses of those patients?"

"Yes."

"Was any such evidence of the strep infection found in Michelle's case?"

"No," Dr. Sogg replied.

Even though Dr. Sogg had been a student of Plaintiffs' expert, Dr. Bettman, while pursuing his specialty in Ophthalmology at Stanford Medical School, and both were on the teaching faculty at the time of trial, he did not hesitate to deny a conversation concerning Michelle's case previously testified to by Dr. Bettman. The two had casually run into one another on campus wherein they entered into a conversation specifically concerning Michelle's case. Dr. Bettman had testified that during this conversation Dr. Sogg told him that the "Pill" could not be ruled out, but he (Dr. Sogg) would hate to see it go that way. Again, the element of bias raised its ugly head.

Compelled from their own entries in the hospital medical records, all three of these treating doctors conceded on cross-examination that thrombosis played a substantial role in Michelle's blindness. Dr. Kosmin and Dr. Lippe could not explain the blindness from infection alone or otherwise. Dr. Sogg chose to blame infection from a cut finger, even though he didn't know if the "Pill" caused clotting. None could produce a similar case from the medical literature or from experience and two admitted none exists. And all three of the treating doctors had previously agreed to testify as expert witnesses for Ortho against their own patient, Michelle, including one of them who at the time of trial had become a product liability consultant for a drug manufacturer.

Although I did not think of it at the time, I later suspected they were also concerned they could be implicated in causing Michelle's blindness for not starting anti-coagulant therapy much sooner, i.e., when clotting was first recognized thirteen hours earlier than when the anti-coagulant therapy was actually started. In short, a conscious or sub-conscious self-defense mechanism could well have been at work within their minds.

As we left the courthouse for the day, Michelle commented, "Sal, on one of my office visits to Dr. Sogg I told him I felt the 'Pill' caused my illness and blindness and that I contemplated suing. He told me, 'I don't believe that at all. That 'Pill' had nothing to do with your blindness.'"

"Well, he sure changed his tune on cross-examination."

As we parted ways with Dennis and Michelle, I turned to Harold, "I think we had another good day. Good job on cross-examination."

"I think you're right, Sal, we got lucky."

CHAPTER 10
Big Pharma Fires Its Big Guns

Harold and I returned to Court the next day feeling we had overcome a major hurdle in not being devastated by the testimony of the treating doctors. Now we could focus on the "hired guns" that Ortho would present as its experts, as well as their in-house witnesses. We agreed that I would take over the remaining cross-examinations.

Bruce Ostler, M.D.

Marion had duly advised the previous day that Dr. Ostler would be their next witness. We had depositions on him taken by plaintiff trial lawyers in previous cases. Harold had also cross-examined him and observed his trial testimony demeanor in another case, so he was able to help me prepare to take him on.

❦

The morning started with Marion announcing: "Your honor, we call Dr. Bruce Ostler to the witness stand."

Marion directed Dr. Ostler to inform the jury of his medical education and expertise. He testified that he was a board-certified ophthalmologist and described how he taught courses at Stanford Medical School under the supervision of our Plaintiffs' expert, Dr. Bettman—an unusual situation to deal with in a jury trial. Dr. Ostler testified that in preparation for his testimony, he had reviewed 180 articles from the medical literature and personally surveyed 223 doctors on the subject of streptococcal orbital cellulitis. Marion then went directly to a key issue in the case.

"Dr. Ostler, he asked, "Do you have an opinion on whether the 'Pill' caused blood clotting or thrombosis in Michelle?"

"Yes, I do not believe it did. Despite the admitted presence of thrombosis in Michelle, I cannot consider the oral contraceptive as a causative factor to thrombosis in Michelle, or in any case . . . I do not believe the 'Pill' predisposes to or causes thrombosis at all in anyone."

"Doctor, what do you believe was the cause of blindness in Michelle?"

"The mechanism of blindness in Michelle was caused solely by infection. It all started with a sore throat, pharyngitis."

"Can you explain why there was no evidence of a sore throat until thirty hours after the onset of her illness?" Marion asked.

Dr. Ostler replied, "Even though I think Dr. Gossack must be a very competent doctor, I think he did very well here, but he took a faulty throat culture when he first saw her."

He conceded there was never absolute positive proof of strep in her throat. To justify his contention of the faulty throat culture, he relied upon an abandoned medical theory in vogue prior to antibiotics in the 1940's in an attempt to explain why Dr. Gossack's swab of the throat cultured negatively. His testimony then took on a stretch beyond reason. He testified about cases of erysipelas (St. Anthony's Fire of the Civil War days) causing bilateral blindness through the mechanism of a strep infection (occurring mostly in the 1800's prior to antibiotics, hot running water and soap).

On cross-examination, I took Dr. Ostler head on:

"Dr. Ostler, is it your opinion under oath to this jury that Michelle had erysipelas?"

"No," he quickly admitted. I believed he suddenly realized he had made a huge mistake by adopting this ancient theory.

"Doctor, are any of these complications of erysipelas even seen in this day and age?"

"No," he quickly replied again with a hint of embarrassment.

Defense witnesses and treating doctors, Dr. Sogg and Dr. Lippe, had also previously agreed in their cross-examination that Michelle did not have erysipelas.

I further inquired, "Doctor, isn't it true that not a single case of bilateral blindness showed up in any of the 180 articles you told us you had researched in preparation for your testimony here today?"

He reluctantly replied, "That's true."

"Nor in your personal survey of 223 doctors?"

"That's also true."

"Further, isn't it true that orbital cellulitis did not exist until Michelle began to show signs of swelling of the eye, after she had appeared in the emergency room?"

"Yes."

"Do you agree that pharyngeal swelling [in the area of the throat] could result from thrombophlebitis of the pterygoid plexus?"

"Yes," again he agreed.

"Isn't it further true that Michelle did have thrombophlebitis throughout her facial veins as one of the early symptoms associated with her early swelling?"

"That is what the records show," he said rather quietly.

"Wouldn't the tenderness in the neck identified by Dr. Gossack on February 15th be consistent with thrombophlebitis of the jugular vein?"

"It would," he replied.

He went on to agree that thrombophlebitis of the facial veins can create a venous backup and thereby cause increased cranial pressure, and white blood cell count of 17,800 (Michelle's when she entered emergency) can occur from thrombosis alone, without infection.

A key question and answer followed:

"Diagnosis of orbital cellulitis and cavernous sinus thrombosis are often mistaken and reversed, isn't that true?"

"I agree," he replied.

Most significant in his cross-examination testimony was when he professed no expertise in clotting problems and deferred to a hematologist the question of the effect of predisposition to clotting, when triggered by an infectious disease. Yet, he still clung to his opinion that the "Pill" did not cause blood clotting or thrombosis in anyone, nor did it create a predisposition for such.

If a medical doctor does not believe the "Pill" causes or predisposes to thrombosis in any case, how could such an expert be objective on the issue of causation in this case? There was the evidence from Alice, Michelle's friend who was with her the day of the onset of her illness and Dennis, negating infection until thirty hours after the onset of the illness. They further indicated symptoms consistent with thrombosis (left sided headache and tender neck). These facts from lay witnesses contradicted the assumptions of a sore throat and a history of infection. Ortho's expert witnesses ignored this evidence, even though known to them from the medical records, the depositions of lay witnesses, and the deposition of Dr. Gossack, all available to them from Ortho. Every expert witness for the Defense testified having never seen a case like it. The uniqueness of this case, if viewed from solely an infection etiology, renders the infection theory alone suspect, if not totally improbable.

After I announced, "No further questions, your Honor," Marion tried to rehabilitate his witness, with little success in the face of the admissions he had given us. Dr. Ostler was another witness who demonstrated how the truth can surface under a strong cross-examination.

Before Dr. Ostler was excused, another intelligent question came from the jury:

"Dr. Ostler, will an inactive strep infection become active in the presence of thrombosis and do you believe the infection here was secondary?"

This resulted in the following admission from Dr. Ostler:

"If thrombosis is associated with the 'Pill' in Michelle's case, an active infection could possibly work in combination with the 'Pill' to lead to thrombosis, which then reactivates the streptococcus by creating a new growth."

In other words, when blood clots in the veins, it often creates the pooling of blood at the clotting site which is a perfect medium for infection to grow. This testimony echoed the opinions earlier stated by Plaintiffs' expert, Dr. Altshuler.

Another juror questioned Dr. Ostler, "In your survey of doctors, did you talk to each of the 223 doctors yourself?"

Dr. Ostler responded, "Of course, this was not possible."

As we left the courthouse after a full day of Dr. Ostler's testimony, Harold and I again related to one another what had become a repeated familiar comment between us, "It was another good day." Michelle and Dennis, however, were having their apprehensions as they listened to testimony from these Defense experts, but indicated some relief after hearing the cross-examination.

WILLIAM McCABE, M.D.

Several more critical Defense witnesses remained, one of them, the next witness, Dr. William McCabe. Since Harold had obtained enough information on him, as well as a transcript of his testimony in another "Pill" case, I didn't feel compelled to incur the expense and time to depose him.

At the beginning of the trial in Ortho's opening statement, while telling the jury about the expert witnesses Ortho would present in the case, Marion had boasted about Dr. McCabe's credentials, and particularly his experience in having performed more than a thousand surgeries on the human skull. He touted Dr. McCabe as one of the most knowledgeable doctors in the world on the anatomy of the human head. Marion claimed that with his unusual knowledge and expertise, he would be able to explain why infection, and not thrombosis, was the sole cause of Michelle's blindness.

I entered the courtroom the next day feeling comfortable that I could handle Dr. McCabe in cross-examination, but could not possibly anticipate what ultimately would happen that day.

"Your Honor, the Defense will call Dr. William McCabe to the stand," Marion proudly announced. Dr. McCabe described his educational background followed by his board certification as an ENT [ear, nose and throat] specialist. He testified that he practiced in his specialty for several years in the State of Iowa.

Dr. McCabe surprisingly admitted he had no expertise in blood clotting, susceptibility to clotting, or in drugs that cause clotting. He would defer those areas to a clotting expert. He did not know if the "Pill" caused clotting or a susceptibility to clotting.

"That's really outside my expertise," he said.

On direct examination, Dr. McCabe displayed significant arrogance and egotism, even for an expert physician.

Dr. McCabe went on to describe a mechanism of blindness, with a few strange similarities to the testimony of Plaintiffs' expert witnesses. "The illness," he said, "began with a strep throat, followed by thrombophlebitis of the *pterygoid plexus*, which then by retrograde thrombophlebitis involved the orbit of the eye." Thereafter, "the infection moved into the orbit causing orbital cellulitis. Intra-orbital pressure then developed and equaled the perfusion pressure of the central retinal artery causing the artery to collapse, thereby starving the blood supply to the retina, resulting in blindness."

He offered that, ". . . without thrombophlebitis of the pterygoid plexus, she would not have developed orbital cellulitis or the blindness." He explained, "the infection [septicemia] came secondarily *from the throat directly to the pterygoid plexus*, then onward to the eyes and orbits. " The last part of his explanation seemed strange to me considering it was coming from a highly competent expert on the anatomy of the head, but I was pleasantly surprised by the mechanism of injury he had so clearly explained on direct examination.

My first question on cross-examination:

"Doctor, do I understand your testimony correctly that you are saying the strep went directly *from the throat to the pterygoid plexus* [behind the cheek bone]?"

Without hesitation, he responded, "Absolutely!"

Dr. McCabe became quite condescending toward me at that point. Here is where he opened himself up to a crucial impeachment. I knew his description was wrong since the pterygoid plexus is located behind the cheek and not in the throat area, having observed it with my own eyes in autopsy only a few months earlier.

Pulling up the collar of my coat, I said, "Doctor, I apologize for my ignorance of medicine as I am just a country lawyer. Would you tell me and the jury where in the human skull is the pterygoid plexus located?"

For those readers who are old enough to remember, in the early 70's there was a popular TV series featuring a smart detective, "Colombo." He always played dumb as a technique when questioning guilty people, and always wore an overcoat with the collar pulled fully up. I was confident the jury recognized exactly who I was mimicking and why. By this time the jury had heard me utilize extensive medical knowledge in both my direct and cross-examinations for several weeks, so I was confident they would realize I was doing this to play on the witness' arrogance, and not on them.

Turning to the jury to observe their reactions, I waited for his response.

He quickly stated with an air of confidence and increased arrogance, "Behind the throat, as I told you."

I then repeated in a humble manner, "Doctor, again I apologize. I am just a lawyer, but are you *sure* the pterygoid plexus is located behind the throat?"

This time he retorted, not only condescendingly, but very emphatically and with anger that I or anyone would ever question his superior knowledge of the anatomy of the human head.

"Certainly, it is located behind the throat, I have seen it a thousand times!"

At this point I walked back from standing near the jury to the counsel table where Harold was sitting. I bent over and whispered so the jury would not hear me, "Harold, I know he is wrong, but refresh my memory on the name of the plexus of veins that is located behind the throat that appear similar to the pterygoid plexis?"

Harold whispered so it could not be heard by anyone in the court room, "the *pharyngeal* plexus."

I returned to stand near the jury, but slightly to their rear. The jury's eyes locked on me anxiously awaiting my next question. I raised my coat collar a little bit higher and turned to watch the jury's reaction as I asked the question again.

"Doctor, please excuse my ignorance of anatomy, but where is the *pharyngeal* plexus located?"

As I was looking at the jury, they had moved to the edge of their seats while locked in a glaring stare at Dr. McCabe anxiously awaiting his response. There was stark silence from the witness stand. Slowly smiles began to appear upon their faces. I turned to look at Dr. McCabe who was sitting with his head faced down, crimson red with embarrassment.

"Doctor, I apologize, but I don't think I or the jury heard your answer?"

While the jury and I waited for what felt like several seconds of silence, a very long time, all of us staring right at him, mumbled words finally emitted from his mouth in a low shallow tone.

"Behind the throat."

Right after the words tumbled out of Dr. McCabe's mouth, Judge Allen unexpectedly, untimely, and clearly interrupting my cross-examination, declared a fifteen-minute recess. Everyone in the courtroom recognized Judge Allen wanted to allow Dr. McCabe an opportunity to compose himself from the embarrassing situation he had self-created. Having touted his expertise on the anatomy of the human skull, he suddenly realized that he had mistaken the pharyngeal plexus located in the throat, from the pterygoid plexus located higher up in the skull in the area of the cheek bone. He knew if infection did originate in the throat, it would have first infected the pharyngeal plexus.

༄

Upon his return to the witness stand, Dr. McCabe's demeanor and testimony was no longer arrogant and even became somewhat respectful. As I continued my cross-examination I asked, "Dr.

McCabe, if one has a predisposition to clotting, is it more likely that an infection will cause thrombosis or thrombophlebitis?"

"That probably is true," he conceded.

"If, in Michelle's case, a susceptibility to clotting is assumed, wouldn't that susceptibility make it more probable for a simple strep throat to lead to thrombophlebitis of the pterygoid plexus?"

"I would defer the mechanism of infection causing thrombosis to a hematologist," he responded.

"Is thrombosis in the pterygoid plexis from a sore throat really something you have commonly seen?"

"Thrombosis in the pterygoid plexis from a sore throat is not common in my experience, only possible, but again, I would defer to a hematologist as the proper specialist on that question."

Further corroborating Plaintiffs' experts on cross-examination, Dr. McCabe agreed with all of the following: that ten days after the onset, Michelle had blocked ophthalmic veins which drain into the cavernous sinus. If thrombophlebitis comes first causing swollen tissue, the situation is ripe for infection and produces a wild, tremendous fulminating infection. Even after the infection was resolved, swelling in Michelle continued due to thrombosis. Thrombosis and not streptococcus (strep) caused the white blood cell count to rise back to 17,700 eleven days later. If infection were the cause, soreness in the throat would come first followed by fever, usually two to six hours later, (none of which occurred in that time frame in Michelle). Redness in the throat would appear fairly early (which also did not happen to Michelle).

"Dr. McCabe, if an examining physician did not see redness, and the throat was not painful and sore, would you agree that there probably was neither a sore throat nor a strep throat in Michelle?"

"Yes, I agree."

Since Dr. Gossack had found no redness or signs of a sore throat when he examined Michelle before hospitalizing her, this admission by Dr. McCabe further substantiated our witnesses' testimony that thrombosis and not infection was the major contributing factor to Michelle's blindness.

Dr. McCabe, voluntarily offered, "I see more cellulitis and cavernous sinus thrombosis than physicians in other parts of the country. I have seen at least forty-five such cases of such."

"Have you seen even a single case develop into bilateral blindness?" I asked.

"This is a rare and unusual case. The bilateral blindness is unique to anything I have seen and is hard to reconcile with orbital cellulitis."

Dr. McCabe, as Ortho's last retained expert on the issue of the cause of Michelle's blindness, thereby nullified his theory of infection as the sole cause, contrary to his earlier testimony on direct examination.

"Dr. McCabe, do you believe that the strep entered Michelle's bloodstream from the cut finger she experienced two weeks earlier?"

"No, that makes no medical sense."

This testimony directly contradicted Dr. Sogg's contention of a cut finger as a portal of entry. Marion's attempt on redirect to improve McCabe's image as an expert accomplished little.

Upon the completion of Marion's redirect of Dr. McCabe, Judge Allen invited the jury to ask questions. Among them, one juror asked a rather hilarious question in light of the previous testimony of Dr. McCabe, "Doctor, did you ever have strep throat?"

He embarrassingly responded affirmatively.

Miss Yue

Marion then advised the Court, "Your Honor, we have one more short witness before we end the day.

"Proceed with your next witness." Judge Allen said.

"The Defense calls Miss Yue to the stand."

Marion had her testify to her expertise as a laboratory technician who was involved in the testing of Michelle's blood with the finding of strep in her blood. She described in detail the laboratory procedure she utilized. As we listened, Harold whispered to me that he didn't feel she was giving an accurate description. At that point, we couldn't be certain of her inaccuracy, but Harold was quite uncomfortable with what he heard. We therefore passed on cross-examining her. She was otherwise uneventful.

∽

Even though it was only early on a Friday afternoon, Judge Allen recessed early advising us to return at 10 a.m. the following Monday. As we left the Courtroom chatting with Michelle and Dennis about their thoughts on the testimony that day, they conveyed their impressions that no one should believe the testimony of Dr. McCabe. He completely lacked credibility. Dennis commented that he immediately picked up on my Columbo act and thought it worked well on the witness.

Dennis and Michelle were feeling much more confident now that they had seen a significant part of the Defense case fall apart. By this point of the trial they both had become quite angry toward Johnson & Johnson, fully convinced they had taken on a justifiable cause. In their minds, they were absolutely convinced this was a worthy battle for the good of society. I agreed with Michelle and Dennis and was proud to be a part of this battle to reach the truth.

That thrombosis and possibly infection together were involved in the mechanism causing Michelle's blindness should no longer have been an issue for the jury. So too, that the "Pill" rendered Michelle more susceptible to thrombosis was clearly established by the foregoing evidence.

Now Ortho (Johnson & Johnson) had to rebut Plaintiffs' contention that they knew or should have known that the "Pill" would cause clotting in some women and failed to warn of that fact. In short, convince the jury they didn't know or even suspect the "Pill" could cause thrombosis.

☙

Harold and I returned to the office that afternoon and Harold called Dr. Altshuler to discuss with him the laboratory procedure described by Miss Yue. Dr. Altshuler informed Harold that before testifying at trial, he had called Miss Yue and spoke with her about the procedure she used. The procedure she described to Dr. Altshuler varied from what she testified to on the stand and opened the door for a possible misdiagnosis as to the existence of a strep infection at all. Dr. Altshuler indicated that he would be willing to return to testify if we felt it was necessary.

ERNEST PAGE, M.D.

As I did my routine evening walk, I pondered what more could Johnson & Johnson possibly throw at us that we were not prepared to deal with? I began to think about how to deal with the expert Marion had designated for Monday, Dr. Page. He too, like others, was a regular expert for Ortho in previous cases, so I had access to his previous testimony to prepare which gave me excellent insight as to what he would be saying on the stand. I knew he would be limiting his testimony to opinions on *warnings only* as given by Ortho, and not causation of Michelle's blindness. We were over the hump on that issue.

Marion had also advised us, before leaving Court, of the possibility of putting another witness on the stand that completely caught us by surprise, none other than the famous Dr. Goldzeirher. When Harold and I heard his name mentioned, we were both quietly ecstatic. My strategy to force them to bring him to trial for fear of hiding evidence worked. We spent the weekend preparing my cross-examination solely on the pre-market and post-market testing documentation as well as the warnings issues for which we had ample ammunition.

∽

Monday morning, Harold and I entered the courthouse, meeting up with Michele and Dennis. They were curious as to what to expect that day. I told them they would get a glimpse of the effects on doctors of the fraudulent conduct of Ortho.

Marion called his next witness, "Your Honor, the Defense calls Dr. Ernest Page to the stand." He began the usual initial testimony of qualifying him as an expert on the issues he would address in his testimony. Dr. Page explained he was an experienced practicing OB-GYN for many years from San Francisco, California (only 50 miles north of our courthouse in San Jose). As an OB-GYN, he described how he has prescribed the oral contraceptive thousands of times with no serious consequences.

I listened to that scenario, reflecting on the fact that when a woman suffered a stroke or heart attack while on the "Pill," she would call emergency, not her OB-GYN. Michelle's case was somewhat exceptional in that regard.

He admitted in his direct testimony that he had never seen Michelle's medical records, had not discussed the case with any physician, and was not going to render any opinion on causation of Michelle's blindness. His focus was going to be solely on the adequacy of the warnings issued by Ortho on the "Pill."

These warnings were limited to stating there was merely a "statistical significant association" between the "Pill" and thrombophlebitis. That was the warning language recommended by the FDA OB-GYN Advisory Committee in 1968, heavily influenced by Johnson & Johnson. There was absolutely no warning of a *cause and effect* relationship. Even that warning, "a statistical significant association," because of delay in publication did not reach the prescribing physician until the early 1970's and certainly had not reached Dr. Gossack or any of Michelle's treating physicians at that time. Dr. Page contended that warning of a "statistical significant association" between the "Pill" and thrombophlebitis, was adequate at the time based upon what was known to the medical world. He stressed how thrombophlebitis can occur spontaneously in women making it more difficult to establish a cause and effect relationship.

I began my cross-examination by asking, "Doctor, have you been provided by Ortho any of the pre-marketing studies on the 'Pill?'"

"No."

"Are you aware of the many adverse reaction reports, including challenge and response cases that had been reported to Ortho and contained in their records?"

"No."

"Doctor, hasn't Ortho offered you access to any of this research material within their own records?"

"No, they haven't."

"Did you ask Ortho to provide you any of such information?"

"No."

"Did Ortho ever tell you of the influence they brought upon the FDA's OB-GYN Advisory Committee to prevent a "cause and effect relationship" warning from being placed in the PDR [Physicians' Desk Reference], and being given to physicians and the public?"

"I am not aware of any such thing occurring," he claimed.

Dr. Page's opinion that the warnings were adequate could not overcome the unimpeachable testimony of the FDA Commissioner, Dr. Ley, or that of Dr. McCleery, whose primary expertise as an FDA staff member focused on the adequacy of warnings to physicians. Nor could it overcome the deliberate falsification by Ortho such as the stroke case reported to Ortho by Dr. Overton. Ortho falsely reported to the FDA that the victim of the stroke had a full recovery, without even checking with Dr. Overton, her treating physician.

Dr. Page also could not explain Ortho's failure to report to the FDA, the triple challenge and response case reported by Dr. Harris. When shown the patient booklet emphasizing the safety of the "Pill" he could give no reasonable explanation for such representation.

As my cross-examination was coming to an end, I sought to explore Dr. Page's deeper thoughts or any opinions he failed to render.

I asked, "Doctor, is it your belief that there is absolutely no cause and effect relationship between the 'Pill' and thrombosis?"

"There might be a cause and effect relationship between the 'Pill' and thrombosis."

"Would you agree then, that the 'Pill' possibly predisposes some women, not all, to thrombosis?"

"Yes, you're probably correct, particularly those with non-O type blood such as A, B, and AB," he conceded.

"Doctor, would you recommend the 'Pill' for a woman who has already experienced thrombosis while on the 'Pill?'"

"I would not prescribe the 'Pill' for a woman who previously experienced thrombosis while on the 'Pill.'"

In the last few answers on cross-examination, Dr. Page provided a bonus that could not possibly have been anticipated. Their own witness admitting causation to some extent. He was no help to Ortho's case but rather, raised more questions than answers with regard to Ortho's failure to adequately warn.

At the completion of Dr. Page's testimony, Judge Allen asked the jurors if they had any questions. Among the questions asked was the following by a juror, "Dr. Page, do you report any adverse reactions, from drugs, that you see in your patients to the drug companies?"

Dr. Page's response was noncommittal.

Michelle and Dennis met us outside the courtroom at the break and they could not believe how weak this Ortho witness' testimony appeared, especially after cross-examination which refreshed the jurors' memory on the powerful contrary testimony by the FDA commissioner, and FDA Staff member, Dr. McCleary.

JOSEPH GOLDZEIRHER, M.D.

In any trial the parties are required to provide the Court with a list of the witnesses, and specifically the retained expert witnesses they intend to have testify. Strangely to Harold and I, missing from Ortho's list was one very significant name, Joseph Goldzeirher, M.D. He was the endocrinologist from El Paso, Texas who was considered one of Ortho's primary investigators in the pre-market testing of the "Pill."

During our three-week discovery trip to Ortho's home office in Raritan, we had obtained substantial evidence of negligent pre-marketing testing, and intentional conduct to minimize the discovery of adverse reactions to the "Pill," including thrombotic events. Our only means of authenticating and introducing these documents into evidence with explanatory testimony would be through cross-examination of Dr. Goldzeirher. Since Dr. Goldzeirher's clinic in El Paso was among the most flagrant in violation of an ethical study, we had hoped Ortho would produce him.

His absence from the list was not surprising to us. Testimony given in other cases demonstrated Dr. Goldzeirher to be a poor witness, unprofessional in his demeanor, and unpredictable in his testimony, even with a lot of preparation. He would be a risk for Ortho on the witness stand in a significant case such as this. We could not subpoena him because he resided out of state. We had not taken his deposition because we assumed Ortho would be compelled to place him on the stand to explain the adequacy of their testing. We also had ample testimony on him from previous trials.

Once we realized he was not on their witness list, we implemented a strategy to create a necessity for Ortho to bring him to testify. At the beginning of the trial, in my opening statement, I emphasized to the jury the importance of Dr. Goldzeirher's clinical studies in determining whether thrombosis was a risk of the "Pill" before it was ever put on the market. Wherever it was pertinent, I emphasized the importance of Dr. Goldzeirher's studies and the interpretation of those studies. I also made sure Dr. Goldzeirher's name was brought up during trial so often that the jury would surely think Ortho was trying to hide something if he were not brought in to testify on his clinical studies.

The strategy worked. Near the end of the presentation of their case Ortho asked Judge Allen if they could be allowed to bring Dr. Goldzeirher into Court to testify on his El Paso Clinical studies. We, of course, did not object. Judge Allen then ordered he could testify.

The Defense prepared him to testify as well as they could. Marion had him set forth his qualifications, not only as to his medical education and practice, but also as a director of clinical studies. Marion focused on Dr. Goldzeirher's clinic as the reason Ortho's Dr. Cronk retained him to carry out its most important pre-marketing clinical studies. Dr. Goldzeirher described his unusually large clinic population he had available for the study, one of the largest in the Unites States at that time. He emphasized that because of the large number of women in his study, if there was any indication the "Pill" was a risk for blood clotting, it definitely would have surfaced.

He elaborated on how not a single case of thrombosis occurred among his substantial clinical patient population over the couple of years of his study, and therefore there was no evidence the "Pill" caused blood clotting of any sort. He concluded his direct testimony by contending there was *no thrombosis risk* to warn about based upon his extensive studies.

I began cross-examination by introducing myself. "How do you do, Dr. Goldzeirher. My name is Sal Liccardo and we have never met before, is that correct?"

"That is true," he said with arrogance.

"Doctor how much has Ortho paid you for your work as an investigator and director of their clinical study on the oral contraceptive?"

"I don't know," he answered without any hesitation.

"Well, can you give us a rough estimate?"

"No."

"It certainly was a substantial amount of money, isn't that true?

"If you say so, I don't recall how much they paid me."

I then handed Marion a three-page document we had obtained from Ortho's records on our discovery trip to Raritan, to review as required before placing it before the witness. Marion scanned it briefly to ensure it was truly an authentic Ortho document.

I then asked the Court, "Your Honor, may I have this marked as Exhibit 201, and may I show it to the witness?"

The Court turned to Marion to see if there was an objection from the Defense. Ortho's personnel did not give any attention to this document when we copied it at their plant. They obviously were completely unaware of all of its contents, to my pleasant surprise.

Seeing that it was properly addressed to Dr. Cronk, Ortho's medical director, "No objection, your Honor," Marion replied. I then placed the document before Dr. Goldzeirher.

"Doctor, please look at the front and the last pages of this three-page document and tell us if you recognize it as a letter from you to Dr. Cronk, the Medical Director at Ortho, soliciting Ortho to retain you and your clinic to perform the early FDA required pre-marketing testing of Ortho-Novum on the childbearing age women who used your health clinic."

He took a few moments to glance at the document.

"Yes, that's my signature on the last page."

"Doctor would you please turn to page two of the letter and please read it out loud to the jury?"

It became apparent that up to that moment he still did not recall what he had written. He began to read aloud the entire page until halfway down where he began to stutter and choke up as he read the following words:

"My clinic will provide for Ortho an ideal medical clinic for a study of the effectiveness and safety of your oral contraceptive. My clinical patient population is very large and diverse *primarily composed of poor, illiterate Mexicans and white trash which will minimize any reporting of side effects from the contraceptive pill.*"

I turned my head and glanced at the jurors as he read that language. Their facial expressions said it all as their immediate shock and anger became apparent. It appeared to me that any credibility Ortho may have had with the jury, as to the integrity of pre-marketing studies, suddenly evaporated.

After an intentional pause on my part, I continued cross-examination focusing on entries from his actual studies demonstrating the total lack of follow-up if a patient stopped coming to the clinic. No attempt was made to find the reasons for the patient not showing up for the next pill. I directed his attention to each patient who had never completed the study and asked:

"Why didn't she show up for her next pill? Did she suffer a stroke, heart attack, thrombophlebitis?"

"I don't know."

"Did she die, Doctor?"

"I don't know," was the response I got over and over as I took him through entry after entry of women who failed to complete the study, without any follow-up to determine the reason for these women dropping out. The loss to follow up patients were more than sufficient to coverup a blood clotting risk.

Where there was follow-up, the reports of the medical findings were so vague, inconclusive, and incompetent as to the complaints, symptoms or illnesses that they were virtually useless to uncovering any risk.

I had him point out from their own records where they would give the monthly prescription of the "Pill" to the patients, husband, sister, brother, or mother without ever seeing the patient herself. In short, this evidence proved the studies by Dr. Goldzeirher to be completely lacking the competence and professionalism necessary to determine if any risk existed in taking the "Pill," especially thrombosis. The very nature of the list of symptoms that his workers were given to review with the patients in their study was medically useless to uncover any blood clotting event that may have occurred. It appeared in the studies that they did everything possible to cover up any thrombosis risk from being discovered. Dr. Goldzeirher's testimony fulfilled our need to get before the jury the hard evidence of complete inadequacy and incompetency in the manner in which Ortho performed their pre-marketing studies. They were clearly conducted without any regard to uncovering any blood clotting risk.

Judge Allen asked if any jurors had any questions of Dr. Goldzierher, among which was the following by a juror:

"Did you ever see or participate in a challenge and response study?"

Goldzeirher's reply was a simple, "No."

❧

Before leaving the courtroom, Marion advised us the next witness would probably be his last. He planned to call Arnold Cronk, M.D. the Medical Director and, of course, the key spokesperson for Ortho Pharmaceutical Corporation and Johnson & Johnson. I felt we were very lucky that we were able to get the chance to cross-examine Dr. Goldzierher just before Dr. Cronk would be testifying. The credibility damage done to Ortho through that cross-examination was sure to rub off on Dr. Cronk in the juror's eyes. After all, Dr. Cronk selected Dr. Goldzierher to do those studies. This witness would be critical to the case. The pressure was on.

"It was another good day," Harold and I both said on our way out of the courtroom.

I asked Dennis and Michelle what were their thoughts on the day.

"If that doesn't stink!" Michelle remarked. "That this man would stoop so low as to test the drug where he knew these people wouldn't report all their reactions—that's rotten. That they would allow husbands and sisters to come in and pick up the drugs for the next month's cycle without questioning or examining the patient themselves is incredibly incompetent."

ARNOLD CRONK, M.D.

After a heavy evening of preparation, I felt as ready as possible to take on the key figure of the Defense. He would certainly be the most prepared Defense witness, and therefore the most difficult to cross-examine.

As we walked into the courthouse that morning and met up with Dennis and Michelle, I thought to myself how, through the process of the trial itself, they had clearly changed from a strong anti-litigation attitude to a realization that an adversarial trial could be a fantastic tool for uncovering the truth and saving lives. They had now become crusaders for justice.

Marion announced to the Court, "Your Honor, the Defense will call its last witness to the stand, Dr. Arnold Cronk." He then had the witness describe his job position.

"I am a Vice-President and the Medical Director of Ortho Pharmaceutical Corporation, a subsidiary of Johnson & Johnson, Inc."

He then provided his medical background—a medical school graduate, trained in the specialty of Internal Medicine. "As the medical Director of Ortho, I am responsible for all pre-marketing and post-marketing testing of all Ortho's pharmaceutical products, including the oral contraceptive, Ortho-Novum."

His testimony substantiated that his power, authority, and influence within Ortho was tremendous. His fingerprints were all over Ortho's entire history of the development of their oral contraceptive product, Ortho-Novum.

His direct testimony followed in great detail the corporate line of defense. The "Pill" does not cause clotting or create a predisposition for such, and Ortho's warnings in its package inserts, patient booklets, and PDR, were adequate and fully complied with FDA regulations. He, too, came across quite arrogant in his demeanor during this testimony, exhibiting a familiar trait of corporate giants.

In cross-examining Dr. Cronk, I first had him establish that he had sole authority to select and approve all the pre-marketing studies, their locale, and the investigators hired to perform them. He admitted that in addition to Dr. Goldzeirher's clinic on the Mexican border in El Paso, Texas, he had further authorized studies in San Juan, Puerto Rico, and Mexico City, all locations where the patient population would be poor, illiterate, and highly susceptible to loss of follow up.

I handed Marion a letter from Ortho's files to be introduced into evidence. He expressed no objection.

"Dr. Cronk, can you identify this letter as one from Ortho's records?"

"Yes."

"Dr. Cronk, the letter I just handed you and had you read was from a physician in upstate New York offering his OB-GYN medical clinic for pre-marketing testing on the Ortho's oral contraceptive, correct?"

"Yes," he agreed reluctantly.

"And this upstate New York physician describes his clinic population as highly educated, as well as very reliable in following through as participants of a medical study, true?"

"That's correct."

"This upstate New York OB-GYN further explains in his letter how his clinic maintained a long personal medical history on most of its patients, thereby making it easy to follow-up on any drop out from the study, is that accurate?"

"Yes."

". . . and further easy to detect and identify any drug side effects and risks from their product, true Doctor?"

"Yes," he murmured, obviously annoyed knowing what was coming.

"Dr. Cronk, your reply letter to his offer was a polite, 'Thank you, but no thanks!' isn't that true?"

"Yes," his voice dropping.

"And subsequent to that refusal, Dr. Cronk, you accepted Dr. Goldzeirher's El Paso Clinic as more desirable for Ortho's pre-market testing of the oral contraceptive, correct?"

"Yes, I considered that a better choice at the time."

"A few years later, the FDA criticized Dr. Goldzeirher for his unprofessional and unethical work in doing such studies, true?"

"That is true."

Dr. Cronk expressed no opinion on the role of the "Pill" or infection in Michelle. He confined his testimony to the issues of cause and effect between the "Pill" and thrombosis in general, clinical and laboratory testing, marketing, and promotion activities concerning the "Pill."

My cross-examination alone of Dr. Cronk evolved into two days of testimony. Because of his position with Ortho as the Medical Director, he was in a position to be not only knowledgeable, but responsible for much of Ortho's conduct relating to the "Pill." For that reason, he could not claim lack of knowledge or ignorance to any of my questioning.

Through his testimony I was able to establish the following facts: Ortho repeatedly failed to report adequate information to the FDA, particularly reported cases of thrombotic disease. They failed repeatedly to seek pre-clearance from the FDA of advertising, as required by law, such as the "patient booklet" on the "Pill" that was distributed to OB-GYNs to place in their patient waiting rooms for easy access. The patient booklet emphasized that the "Pill" was "safe" without any indication whatsoever of any risk of blood clots, etc., despite studies to the contrary in the late 1960's. It even went so far as to claim that a reliable study from Great Britain on British women, which demonstrated a causal relationship of the "Pill" to blood clotting, was *not applicable to American women.*

"Dr. Cronk, can you tell me what is the difference between British women and American women in their reaction to Ortho-Novum?" I asked.

"I cannot," he embarrassingly conceded.

That false statement in their advertising was specifically in the PDR published to practicing physicians, as well as the Package Insert that accompanied each "Pill" prescription, only to pharmacists at that time.

"Doctor, you are familiar, are you not, with the triple challenge and response case reported to Ortho by Dr. Harris here in Mountain View, who testified to it in this trial?"

"Yes, I am."

"We obtained that information from Ortho's own files, correct?"

"If you say so, yes."

"Didn't you have a duty under the law to report that to the FDA when it came to your attention?"

He murmured almost inaudibly, "Yes."

"But you failed to do that, true?"

"Yes," he softly conceded.

∽

He admitted six challenge and response cases were reported to Ortho, prior to February 1969 (the time of Michelle's illness), and that Dr. Harris's triple challenge and response case was reported to Ortho as early as 1966 (three years before Michelle's blindness). As we previously learned, only one challenge and response case was brought to the attention of Dr. Ley, the FDA Commissioner, prior to late 1969. Dr. Ley had testified that after he had succumbed to the industry position, it was the *multiple challenge and response cases* that provided the evidence to convince him of a cause and effect relationship when he subsequently learned about them, and that the industry cover up of these cases was wrong.

"Dr. Cronk, Ortho was told in May 1968 of a comparable epidemiological study [a study designed to find causation, if it exists] to the British studies on the oral contraceptives conducted within the United States by a Dr. Sartell, true?"

"Yes."

"And Dr. Sartell's study had comparable preliminary findings as the British study?"

"Yes."

"Nonetheless, in Ortho's July 1968 package insert, Ortho stated 'no comparable studies are yet available within the United States.' true?"

"Yes."

"This was a deceptive representation, wasn't it?"

"If you say so."

This deception by Ortho was compounded by the fact that Dr. Cronk conceded many of Ortho's own clinical studies, utilized to obtain FDA marketing approval, were conducted outside the United States, in Mexico, Puerto Rico, the Fiji Islands, and Canada.

Dr. Cronk further conceded that Ortho never informed its own marketing and advertising personnel, including detail men, of existing adverse reaction reports, nor of the need to solicit such information from physicians.

The callous attitude of Ortho towards women's health was evident from his further testimony:

"Dr. Cronk, you received a report of a stroke occurring in a patient of Dr. Overton, in Texas, who testified in this case, do you recall that?"

"Yes," he said reluctantly.

"And your reply to Dr. Overton, a neurosurgeon, was substantially, 'you are on the wrong track doctor, don't go on pursuing this.' Isn't that true?"

Dr. Cronk replied, "I don't recall what I said," clearly not denying having made that callous reply, previously testified to by Dr. Overton. The deliberate suppression of adverse information, and the wanton disregard for the safety of the users of the "Pill" was not lost on this jury.

I obtained verification from Dr. Cronk that Ortho had *destroyed* all records and inter-office memoranda pertaining to the 1968 conferences with the FDA when the "cause and effect" change in the language of the package insert was at issue. Yet, he confirmed that internal sales bulletins predating those years, but favorable to Ortho, were retained even to the time of this trial.

Certain medical journals and literature became affluent with case reports and studies linking the "Pill" to thrombosis in a "cause and effect" relationship as early as 1961 (8 years before Michelle's blindness). Dr. Cronk verified that Ortho's medical library received these journals and appropriate personnel within Ortho were aware of these articles. Ortho was particularly aware of an article by Dr. Walsh in the Archives of Ophthalmology analyzing sixty-nine reported cases, of which twenty or more concerned vascular injuries to the eyes in women on the "Pill," including six challenge and response cases.

Dr. Cronk reluctantly verified receipt by Ortho of a preliminary publication of an epidemiology study by the British in 1967 on morbidity and mortality from *thrombosis*, warning of a causal relationship to the "Pill," but it was ignored in Ortho's own so-called warnings. He conceded that studies establishing a susceptibility to thrombosis in women with type A, B, or AB blood was known to Ortho as early as 1968 as creating a greater risk when on the "Pill." Yet, no mention of this knowledge was ever communicated to prescribing physicians in the package inserts or other published material by Ortho.

Dr. Cronk agreed that case reports linking the "Pill" to thrombosis were received by Ortho as early as 1962, increasing to approximately 300 at the time of trial, including cases of blindness, a few cases of optic neuritis (vascular occlusions in and about the eyes), 6 challenge and response cases, and 50 death cases, many prior to Michelle's blindness. In many cases, thrombosis was reported in unique sites such as the intestine, kidney, auxiliary vein in the arm, abdominal veins, and other unusual areas where thrombosis is not known to occur spontaneously.

That all of the above occurred and was made known to Ortho, before Michelle's blindness, could not be denied by Dr. Cronk. He further confirmed that as early as 1962, Ortho attended a conference sponsored by G.D. Searle & Co., another "Pill" manufacturer, at which many reported thrombosis cases were secretly discussed and reviewed. Ortho and Syntex, another "Pill" manufacturer, agreed to confidentially exchange adverse reaction reports received by each in the same early years. These pharmaceutical manufacturers all used the same estrogen component "ethinyl estradiol" as Ortho.

Despite all of this adverse notice to Ortho, Dr. Cronk conceded that as of the time he was testifying, Ortho still had not warned physicians or the public that a cause and effect relationship existed between the "Pill" and thrombosis. The 1968 recommendation of the FDA OB-GYN Committee to warn of a cause and effect relationship was still being ignored by Ortho six years later, at the time of the *Ahearn* trial in 1974. Despite all of the adverse notice of a causal relationship between the "Pill" and thrombosis, he admitted:

"Doctor, as you sit here today, isn't it true that Ortho's patient booklet designed, published, and distributed by Ortho, is still promoting the 'Pill' as 'safe . . . well tolerated . . . causes only minor discomforts' and further representing to women 'there is no medical evidence whatsoever to substantiate fears of harm from taking the 'Pill.'"

"Yes," he softly murmured.

"And these were the same patient booklets that have never been approved nor cleared by the FDA, despite the requirement of such by Federal Law?"

"I guess that's true," he admitted.

Marion asked very little on redirect examination.

Judge Allen extensively questioned Dr. Cronk before jurors' questions. The nature of the questions emanating from Judge Allen I found perplexing in terms of his understanding of the issues in the case. A sample is as follows:

"These charts talk about the incidence of thrombophlebitis. Can you tell me again what that is?" (The medical glossary provided to the Court and each juror at the beginning of trial contained the definition of thrombophlebitis as well as weeks of testimony on the subject by this time.)

"What does prospective mean?

"Regarding clinic patients lost to follow-up, they might have gone to Africa."

"I assume the jurors are like me. If somebody reads a long document, your mind wanders. . . ."

When Judge Allen finished his questioning, the jurors were invited to ask their own questions. Based on the jurors' questions, there was no doubt the jury saw through Ortho's conduct to minimize the finding of side effects from the "Pill."

The jurors' questions were focused on the studies and lack of communication to the FDA and physicians, such as the following:

"Did any of your studies have matched controls?"

Dr. Cronk replied, "No, because it would be unethical to give women a placebo telling them that it was the 'Pill.'"

When they were finished, Marion announced "Your, Honor, the Defense rests our case."

I arose, "Your Honor, the Plaintiffs would request a recess to allow time to present two rebuttal witnesses."

Judge Allen responded. "We will recess for the day, the jury is excused, and I would like counsel to remain."

All the jurors exited the courtroom.

Judge Allen continued the proceedings addressing me, "Counsel, who are the rebuttal witnesses you intend to call?"

"Your Honor, we would like to call Dr. Bettman back to the stand to rebut the testimony given by Dr. Sogg contending he never said that the 'Pill' could have contributed to Michelle's blindness as alleged by Dr. Bettman in his direct testimony."

The Court replied. "I'm not going to allow Dr. Bettman's rebuttal testimony. Who is the other rebuttal witness you want to call?"

"Your Honor, we would like to call Dr. Altshuler who could be here tomorrow morning to testify in rebuttal of the Defense witness Miss Yue with regard to a discrepancy in her testimony concerning laboratory procedures she used in identifying the strep infection. In preparation for his testimony, Dr. Altshuler had contacted her to confirm that the appropriate laboratory procedures were followed."

Judge Allen said, "I will allow very limited rebuttal testimony on this issue."

He then recessed the Court proceedings for the day.

❧

The following morning, Dr. Altshuler again took the stand to discuss his understanding of the laboratory technical procedures used by Miss Yue from a telephone conversation he had had with her. His testimony appeared to resolve a misunderstanding in communications and amounted to no additional significant evidence in the case.

From our standpoint, however, it was advantageous to have Dr. Altshuler back on the stand as the last witness in the case in that his mere appearance refreshed in the jury's minds the powerful testimony he had rendered a few weeks earlier. This fulfilled our goal of achieving primacy and recency in the presentation of witnesses.

Dr. Altshuler's testimony ended the day and the presentation of evidence at trial. The remainder of the trial days would entail closing arguments by both sides and instructions to the jury on the law applicable to the case. Harold and I left the courthouse convinced that it was another successful day, and that the jury got the message of Ortho's callousness. The jurors' questions to Dr. Cronk the day before confirmed this feeling.

࿇

We met the following day with the Court to review, and get approval on, which instructions of law would be given to the jury. Each side had prepared the instructions it favored, although many were the same. A major conflict occurred when the Defense argued that, under the law, there was no duty at that time to warn the public about a prescription drug, only the physician.

They were correct, as to the law at that time, except for the following exception: I argued that Ortho, in fact, promoted to the public at large through their patient booklet, and therefore, by that act, legally *assumed the duty* to avoid being deceptive or misleading. I argued having assumed that duty to warn, Ortho had a duty not to deceive the public by concealing any known risk. Surprisingly, Judge Allen, agreed with our contention and allowed our instruction on that point to be given to the jury.

We had further discussions with Judge Allen on the wording of the General Verdict form the jury would be required to complete indicating their verdict. Once approved by the Court, each side could refer to any jury instruction, including the verdict form, in their closing arguments to the jury at the close of trial. Judge Allen required that a Special Verdict question be contained within the General Verdict Form as follows:

"*Was Ortho-Novum a substantial factor in bringing about Plaintiff Michelle Ahearn's blindness?*"

This, of course, was the most crucial issue in the entire case.

We then recessed until the next day when I would argue the case to the jury. Harold and I discussed the details of opening argument I would make, referred to formally as summation. As always, that is a long tough night of preparation.

CHAPTER 11
SUMMING UP THE TRUTH

Summation is the first opportunity for the lawyers on each side to argue, not only the facts of their case, but how the law applies to those facts. The plaintiffs are given the opportunity to present the first summation (opening argument) solely because they, and not the Defense, have the burden of proof under the law.

On the morning of December 11, 1974, as Harold, Dennis, Michelle and I entered the courtroom, I was surprised to discover the spectator gallery was almost packed. Word of the timing of final arguments had spread through the local legal profession in that a large part of the audience were lawyers as well as several members of the press. This was an unusual case for Santa Clara County at the time.

As we reconvened trial proceedings, Judge Allen addressed me.

"Counsel are you prepared to proceed with your opening argument?"

"Yes, your Honor."

I arose and walked up to the front of the jury box, turned slightly toward the Judge's bench.

"May it please the Court, my worthy adversaries, and ladies and gentlemen. This is now my opportunity to address you directly on the law and the evidence. Let me first begin by thanking you for your continuous attention and focus during this entire seven weeks of trial. It has been obvious from your questions of the various witnesses that you are a very conscientious jury and are here to do the right thing.

"Further, we all appreciate that this is a great sacrifice of your time taken away from personal matters and work. Let me also apologize for the lengthy jury selection process, however, I know you will appreciate and realize its necessity once you are in the jury room deliberating this case.

"Let me now review with you some of the law that will guide you in your interpretation of the evidence. You are here, as the judge of the facts, to reach a *verdict*—a word derived from Latin meaning *to speak the truth*. You are here to speak the truth in Michelle's case. Only nine of the twelve of you jurors are required under the law to agree on the verdict."

I began a discussion of the law that Judge Allen would include in his final instructions following closing arguments and how it would apply to this case.

"As judges of the facts you should use your common sense to decide who is telling the truth and who isn't, who is biased, and who isn't, and the motivations behind that person's testimony. You will use your conscience to speak the truth. You will be saying either, on the one hand, that Ortho manufactured a pill that does not cause clotting or did not cause clotting in Michelle's case. And that this was the result of the most common bug in the world, strep, which is experienced by every human being in their lifetime. You will be saying that Ortho adequately warned doctors and women—if you reach a Defense verdict.

"On the other hand, you will be saying that the 'Pill' was a *substantial factor* in causing her blindness, and further, that Ortho never warned her doctor or her that there was this risk, if you reach a verdict for Michelle—the truth.

"In a civil case, such as this, Michelle and Dennis, as the Plaintiffs, have the burden to prove by a *preponderance of the evidence* that the 'Pill' was a substantial factor in causing Michelle's blindness, and that Ortho knew, or should have known, that this could happen, yet failed to warn of the risk. 'Preponderance of the evidence' is evidence that has more convincing force than that opposed to it."

I then went up to an easel with a white pad and drew the scales of justice. "Our burden is to tip those scales in our favor ever so slightly by the evidence we presented. In other words, prove our facts by a greater probability of truth—a more likely than not standard. If the evidence is evenly balanced, such that you are unable to say that the evidence on either side of an issue preponderates, then your finding on that issue must be against us, the party who had the burden."

I contrasted the burden of proof required under the law in a criminal case, which is much greater proof—"beyond a reasonable doubt"—because in that situation a human being's freedom or even their life is at stake, and not merely money damages. I then discussed California law on *causation*.

"The Court will instruct you that you must find the 'Pill' was *a proximate cause, a substantial factor* in bringing about Michelle's blindness. However, the law does not require that the alleged cause be the only cause, *the* cause, but can be merely *a cause*. We do not have to prove that Michelle's blindness would not have occurred, but for her being on the 'Pill.' We only have to prove that the 'Pill' was *one of several* factors, but a *substantial* one, that contributed to her blindness. The cause merely needs to be one of several causes, so long as it is *substantial* and not trivial."

Then I applied the foregoing law to the facts of Michelle's case for the jury.

"There exists several possible identifiable contributing causes under the evidence of Michelle's blindness—type "B" blood, strep in her blood stream, thrombosis, and the oral contraceptive. Even the Defense does not dispute that thrombosis was the immediate cause of her blindness. Testimony from both sides agree that thrombosis occurred, backing up the venous flow of blood from the optic nerves. The only question for you to answer is whether the primary initial cause of the thrombosis was infection alone, or in combination with other clotting factors to which Michelle was exposed, such as the 'Pill.' No one disputes that she had type B blood which is a known blood clotting factor. We never disputed that she had a strep infection in her blood [septicemia[, another potential clotting factor, even though no site of the infection could be found. The key question was whether the 'Pill' was *also a substantial factor* in making her more susceptible to blood clotting, 'a sitting duck' in the words of Dr. Bettman and Dr. Altshuler. To reach a verdict for Michelle, all nine of you jurors need *not* agree on the same exact mechanism of causation, but only that the 'Pill' in some way played a significant role—a substantial factor in causing her blindness.

"The legal theories upon which we rested our case of liability are *breach of express warranty, and negligence.* Agreement of nine jurors on either theory or combination, would be sufficient to reach a verdict for Michelle.

"Breach of warranty does not require any negligence. It is an affirmation of fact, or a promise, made by the seller to the buyer and/or her physician which relates to the drug and represents that the drug conforms to the representation, written or oral. Simply put, to say the 'Pill' is 'safe with no serious side effects' is a promise or affirmation. If that is false, there is liability on the seller. Causation—that the 'Pill' caused the injury would still have to be proven.

"Ortho's detail men distributed booklets to doctors to place in their waiting room, so patients could read them while waiting or take them home saying:

> 'Some women have a fear of swallowing any kind of pills, drugs, or medication. They feel all drugs are unnatural and that it might be injurious to their health or somehow affect the children they may have in the future. *There is no medical evidence whatsoever to support these fears.'*

"You have heard that phrase read more than a few times throughout this trial. Such statements by Ortho, ladies and gentlemen, are statements of fact, and if found by you to be untrue, and lead to the purchase and use of Ortho-Novum, Ortho and Johnson & Johnson are liable in this case.

"Other booklets published and distributed by Ortho were intentionally designed to persuade women to take the 'Pill' and expressed or implied no serious risk.

> 'When taken as directed, Ortho-Novum does not interfere with your state of well-being. Discontinue medication pending examination if there is sudden partial or complete loss of vision or if there is sudden onset of proptosis, diplopia or migraine.'

"Was that a helpful warning to Michelle? Once these symptoms develop, as they did in Michelle, it is too late to stop taking the 'Pill.' Michelle had stopped. That is no warning."

I then directed the jury's focus to the package inserts and PDR information disseminated by Ortho to prescribing physicians such as Dr. Gossack, that stated: "Although the following side effects have been reported in users of oral contraceptives, *no cause and effect relationship has been established.*"

"This was the content of the 1967 PDR relied upon by Dr. Gossack, ignoring all the substantial evidence from studies, challenge and response cases, and enormous accumulated evidence known to Ortho by that time establishing a probable cause and effect relationship. Then when you get to the 1968 revised warnings, they no longer mention the phrase that there is *'no cause and effect,'* but rather shift to the confusing phrase, *'statistical significant association'* which as you heard from Dr. Gossack, Dr. Altshuler and even Dr. McCleery of the FDA, was a meaningless term to the prescribing physician. They relate a small part of the British studies which showed a significant risk to thrombosis in that later warning, but then water it down by saying: 'no comparable studies are yet available in the United States'. This was a false statement because they knew by that time that Dr. Sartwell was just completing a comparable study in the United States which confirmed the risk found in the British study. These are false representations of fact by Ortho.

"There is in evidence, ladies and gentlemen, a document that we did not have the opportunity to read to you during Dr. Cronk's cross-examination that I want to call to your attention at this time. This document is an inter-office memorandum of Syntex reciting minutes of a meeting that occurred in April 1, 1968, almost one year before Michelle's blindness, at which all the 'Pill' manufacturers attended, including Dr. Cronk from Ortho. It begins with:

> 'An emergency meeting of the medical directors of all contraceptive manufacturers was called, . . . Dr. Ley [FDA Commissioner at the time] distributed a tabulation of fatal and non-fatal events occurring in association with the use of all contraceptives that have been reported to the FDA for the period from January 1, '66 to December 31, '67. Dr. Ley then informed the meeting that the FDA and its advisory committee have reviewed additional data on thrombophlebitis and pulmonary embolisms that have been received from Great Britain. In their opinion this new data does establish a definite *cause*

and effect relationship between oral contraceptives
and thromboembolic phenomena.'

"In addition to that conclusion of the British scientists studying this
problem, you were read the deposition of Dr. Ley who stated he,
himself, reached this same conclusion before leaving his position
as commissioner at the FDA in 1968, but for whatever reason, did
nothing about it. If thrombosis is occurring spontaneously in these
women who are the subject of so many case reports, why hasn't
thrombosis reoccurred once they are off the 'Pill?' Further, why
does thrombosis occur so often in women on the 'Pill' in places
where it is not known to occur spontaneously, such as blindness
in Michelle?

"The evidence clearly establishes that Ortho made false and
misleading statements in the information they disseminate on the
'Pill.' Prescribing doctors and their patients clearly relied upon
these promises of safety in taking the 'Pill,' including Dr. Gossack
and Michelle. The 'Pill' was at least a *substantial factor* in causing
Michelle's blindness. Thus, the burden of proof that Ortho is liable
for breach of warranty to Michelle has been met by a preponderance
of the evidence as required by law and should support your verdict
for Michelle.

"Let me now discuss with you the legal theory of negligence.

"His Honor will instruct you that: 'The manufacturer of a
drug is under a duty to make adequate warning to the prescribing
physician about the risk and dangers associated with the use of
its product when from the results of animal testing or human use
or other studies it knows or in the exercise of reasonable care
should know that such risks or dangers exist. *Failure to adequately*

warn would be negligence. This duty to warn is a continuing one existing for the period of time that the drug is on the market. The warning should be sufficient to apprise the general practitioner, as well as the unusually sophisticated medical person, of the dangerous propensities of the drug. *That is, it is incumbent upon the manufacturer to bring the warning home to the doctor.'*

"I submit the phrase 'statistical significant association' does not satisfy that criteria of the law. The law further provides that:

> 'A manufacturer of a drug, such as the Defendant here, has a duty to keep abreast of the developments which touch upon its product. It is expected to possess the skill and knowledge of an expert in this field. Although the law provides that compliance with FDA regulations or directives as to the warnings is not negligence. . . when the manufacturer knows of or has reason to know of greater dangers not included in the warning, its duty to warn may not be fulfilled.'

"No mere compliance, ladies and gentlemen, with the FDA is sufficient. The FDA cannot be used as a shield against liability by a pharmaceutical company, any more than the doctor.

"Significantly, the law does not exempt a drug manufacturer from liability just because only a few people are injured by its product. Therefore, the negligence theory of law applicable in this case requires: (1) adequacy of warnings to the physician and the patient. (2) The duty to keep abreast of scientific knowledge. (3) Adequacy of testing before marketing. Dr. Goldzierher's bigoted designation of his clinic population as 'Illiterate, poor, Mexican and white trash,' people who he concedes have no traceable medical history, and further are not easily traced if they drop out of the study, solely to avoid side effects like thrombosis from being discovered, is hardly 'adequate scientific testing.' (4) FDA compliance by itself is insufficient.

"All the foregoing have been violated by Ortho as to warnings as we have previously discussed. The next requirement under the negligence theory is legal causation. That, too, we have fully explored and proven in the evidence presented at this trial.

"We reviewed the evidence of the mechanism by which the 'Pill' causes blood clotting in *some* women. Michelle was double dosed by taking 2 pills within 24 hours as directed by Ortho and her physician. She therefore had ample exposure to clotting from the 'Pill,' which, when added to her susceptibility of having Type B blood, set her up for a disaster once she was exposed to a trigger such as a strep infection."

∾

After summing up all the evidence and witness testimony on the liability issues, I then faced one of my major concerns in the trial. Would I appear to be overreaching to this well-educated jury by asking for damages in the amount I had plead in the original complaint when it was filed, $1 million dollars for Michelle and $250,000 for Dennis?[6] At the time of this trial, in 1974, a verdict of or above a million dollars was exceedingly rare in a personal injury case.

There were less than a couple dozen verdicts for personal injury, or even death in that range, at this time in the United States.

---

6   In 1970 when the complaint was filed, the law required the complaint to contain the amount of damages requested. California law has since removed that requirement.

I mentally agonized over this issue, then finally settled on the following approach:

"I remind you of the testimony of Michelle and Dennis wherein they described that at the time of this catastrophe, Michelle was in good health, 29 years old, happily married housewife for nine years with three small children, ages 2, 5, and 8—a close family. She was a vivacious wife and mother who enjoyed playing sports with her children, golfing, bowling and bridge with her friends, dining, taking long family trips and the ordinary pleasures of life. She was an accomplished pianist, an avid reader, and generally epitomized a happy, normal person. All of this and more has been permanently taken from her by irreversible blindness. In Dennis' words, 'She has lost all of her independence as an individual to be able to function as a mother and a wife to me.'"

Specifically addressing compensation, I continued my argument:

"You will have to decide how you compensate a thirty-five-year-old mother of three small children for spending the rest of her life in absolute darkness—total blindness. The law doesn't give you any fixed standard or formula to apply. You must rely upon your own common sense.

"One part of the damages is simple, the medical bills which total $4,986.00 [remember this is 1969]. His Honor will instruct you that in addition to being compensated for medical expenses, she is entitled to loss of earning capacity. Now, we know Michelle was not working at the time of this catastrophe outside the home. Her work was that of a mother, a housewife to her husband, and taking care of Dennis's secretarial needs in his self-run business as a structural engineer. The law recognizes that there is a real monetary value to what a woman does in her own home even though she is not being paid. This is earning capacity, whether the duties range from baking pies, mopping floors, caring for small children, shopping for groceries, it all has a definite dollar value.

"Think in terms of what would it cost to hire someone to perform each and every chore that Michelle used to be able to do, but no longer can? It would be very expensive to replace any one of you women jurors in your household chores. So, we must look at what are the activities she can no longer do because of her blindness. As you heard from her own testimony there are things she can do, amazingly. You saw her character. She is not the type of person that just gives up trying to do anything because of being blind. Contrarily, she courageously struggles to perform every task she possibly can.

"What can't she do? She can't shop. Someone has to do it for her. She can't select any particular thing in the home or the marketplace. Someone else has to do it for her. When emergencies occur in the house—a child comes running to her crying in pain from an injury, she is helpless to aid that child. In her mind she's saying, is it serious? What do I need to do and how can I do it? Do I need to call the doctor, or does it just need a band-aid? You can go on and on with all the various activities and the things that occur in daily life, and then ask the question—can a blind person handle it? How do you put a price on this loss? What would it cost to replace this loss with outside help?

"I will give you a suggested approach that I believe is reasonable, but it is merely a suggestion. You may have a better one. I believe it would cost much more than $10.00 a day to provide Michelle the daily help she needs. It has to cover a 24-hour period. If in the middle of the night one of her children gets ill, and Dennis is away on business, she needs someone there to help. She starts phoning neighbors looking for help. The total dependency on others is frightening in itself. I think $10.00 a day for the rest of her life for that one element of damages, loss of earning capacity, would not be unreasonable. Her life expectancy based upon mortality tables, as His Honor will instruct you, is 42.2 years. At a mere $10.00 a day, her earning capacity loss would be at today's current market $154,000.00. You may feel she should get $20.00 per day, and if so, just double it. I don't believe that either I or anyone else can tell you what would be reasonable. That is for you to decide.

"His Honor will further instruct you that Michelle is to be compensated for any pain, fears, anxiety, or other mental and emotional distress suffered by Michelle, and of which her injury was a legal cause, and for such sufferings reasonably certain to be suffered in the future from the same cause. We call that *general damages*. I believe this is the major portion of damages Michelle has to live with for the rest of her life. In a civil case the law attempts by money damages to make the injured party whole to the extent possible. Obviously only God could give Michelle back her sight. As jurors you don't have the ability to do that. You can only make her whole by way of money, by way of dollars. The law says if you find Ortho and Johnson & Johnson are liable in this case, then they must compensate her for this loss.

"Now, the above has to be taken together with Michelle's husband, Dennis's situation and loss. He is also a Plaintiff in this case for his individual loss caused by these Defendants. He has stayed very devoted and helpful to her, and from the testimony of both, you know they will stay together for the rest of their lives.

His life expectancy however is less than hers because he is a male, 38.6 years according to mortality tables. That means there is a probability of four years statistically that she won't have Dennis to help her in her blindness. At that time, she will also be up in age and more in need than ever for the support and help from Dennis. This has to be factored in as well when evaluating damages. Here again I think you have to evaluate, as difficult as it is, what is our sight worth to us? How do you compensate someone who has lost it? One way, and again merely a suggested approach, what do we do and how much do we spend to create things that are visually satisfying to us?

"We are entering the Christmas season and as I look around, I see the bright lights going up on homes, Christmas trees, the decorations, everything that is done to create the mood and the atmosphere of happiness and joy. How do you create this mood through these visions to a blind person? She can hear, but she can't see it. She sees blackness. She doesn't see the Christmas lights. How do you do this? You can't.

"Our moods are affected by the weather. If it is a cloudy day, many times many of us get depressed. What must life be like to go through day by day, minute by minute in total absolute blackness? And what effect must that have on a person's mood? Michelle gets up here and laughs and acts very cheerful and it has amazed me to no end, but we know—and as her husband pointed out, the difficulties that this has on her mood, on her anxiety, fears and all those various things that you can't put a finger on that affect and make life worthwhile.

"What people spend just as something extra. They have a home on a seashore so they can have a beautiful view of the sea, pay hundreds of thousands of dollars for that. A prime lot the size of a postage stamp sometimes for that view. The things we do. We go to theaters to see things to satisfy, to get enjoyment and pleasure and affect our mood and our whole lifestyle by what we see and we are spending money galore day in and day out for this.

"When someone has been deprived of this, I think we have to look in terms of all that kind of money being wasted on her. She can't see these things. She has got to be compensated for this loss and that's going to be the most difficult task I think you are going to have in this case; how much to give her for this.

"My feeling, ladies and gentlemen, is that she should be given what we call the prayer. The prayer is the amount that we put in a complaint when we file a lawsuit and it is put in as the upper amount, the limit. And as I have gone through the trial and gone through the case and lived with it for five years, I feel that, though no amount of money would adequately compensate her, she is deserving of the prayer in this case for these general damages and that is *one million two hundred thousand dollars*. And I don't hesitate telling you that, because that I wouldn't take to give up my sight and I am sure Michelle wouldn't either."

Marion quickly and vigorously jumped up objecting at this point stating, "If the Court please, that is not a proper way to measure damages, your Honor, and I think counsel is aware of it."

Judge Allen ruled, "It's argument," then turning to me stated, "Go ahead."

"Thank you, your Honor," I replied, and then continued my summation:

"In addition to Michelle's damages under the law you are allowed, if you see fit, to compensate Dennis for his loss. His Honor will instruct you that under the law you are allowed to compensate Dennis for the value of the services of his wife that have been lost in the past and in the future, if you find liability. It is obvious that there are many things Dennis has to do now that he did not have to do before Michelle's blindness. How much to compensate Dennis for this, again, becomes a difficult task. Time is money in this world we live in, especially to a professional person such as an engineer who gets paid for the time he devotes to his work. The time Dennis now has to spend doing things Michelle use to do before she was blind, doing yard work, shopping for groceries, driving the kids to school, to games, to friends' homes. The lost time all adds up in a lifetime. This time is now taken from the time he would have put into his business working as an engineer. These are thoughts I am going to leave in your hands to consider. You may feel Dennis shouldn't be compensated at all. I leave that solely in your hands, but the law does allow for him to be compensated in this situation for these losses to him. I think Ortho and Johnson & Johnson should be held responsible for all of this loss if justice is to be done. Thank you."

⁓

The Court then recessed for lunch to resume at 1:30 p.m. for Marion to give his summation.

Harold and I gathered with Dennis and Michelle for a few moments. They all expressed how pleased they were with my opening argument. I told them I would need to remain to prepare for my closing argument as they went off to lunch.

⁓

The Court reconvened at 1:30 p.m. Judge Allen stated to Marion, "Counsel you may proceed with your argument."

On behalf of Ortho and Johnson & Johnson, Marion argued that the entire and sole cause of the blindness was due to orbital cellulitis caused entirely by strep. He contended that all three treating doctors, whom they presented in their case, supported that conclusion. Ortho claimed all treating doctors denied the role of the "Pill" as a contributing factor. They admitted the existence of clotting and thrombophlebitis in the orbital and facial veins but attributed it entirely to the strep infection.

Denying that the "Pill" caused clotting in women at all, Ortho contended that thrombosis occurred spontaneously in the population, regardless of the "Pill," relying upon the direct testimony of their experts, as well as the treating doctors, but overlooking the shift in their testimony accomplished on cross-examination. Marion explained away the many adverse reaction reports occurring in the medical literature and described them as spontaneous occurrences of thrombosis, and not in any way related to the "Pill." Relying on the spontaneous occurrence argument, Ortho argued its warnings were therefore adequate in the package insert, the PDR, and the patient booklets, and that under the law they had no further duty to warn.

Ortho argued that the pre-marketing studies performed by their retained medical investigator, Dr. Goldzierher, were more reliable than the British and other studies performed by an independent epidemiologist. Their reasoning was that Ortho's study was prospective (following patients forward), and prospective studies are more scientifically reliable, whereas the published studies were all retrospective (starting with thrombosed or deceased patients and looking backward).

Marion's argument continued for the entire afternoon. At 4:30 p.m. Judge Allen interrupted Marion to recess the jury until 9 a.m. the next morning.

✐

As we left the courthouse, Michelle commented to Harold and me, "Our case is very strong. I can't comprehend how Mr. Pothoven's arguments could possibly nullify all the strong evidence in our favor."

I responded, "I don't like the Defense's argument being split overnight. That not only gives Marion a fresh start in the morning, but also leaves the jury to dwell overnight on his arguments."

We parted for the evening and I returned to my office to work on my closing argument.

✐

The next morning as we entered the crowded courtroom, I had the usual end-of-the-trial good feeling that by the end of this day, I would finally be able to relax and my job would be finished.

Judge Allen took the bench and immediately instructed Marion to continue with his summation. Marion thanked the Judge and continued his arguments on why Ortho-Novum was not proven by a preponderance of the evidence to be the cause of Michelle's blindness, and therefore, that the jury must return a defense verdict despite obvious sympathy for Michelle. He emphasized how difficult it would be to bring in a verdict against Michelle, but justice demanded that they have the courage to do just that.

He reminded the jury of the wonderful history of Johnson &
Johnson and their earned reputation as a pharmaceutical company
producing lifesaving products for many decades. He dwelled on
the tremendous positive value to society contributed by this very
product, Ortho-Novum. He pointed out the millions and millions
of users worldwide thereby controlling the population explosion
throughout the entire world. If this product was so dangerous, why
were not millions of women experiencing thrombosis and dying
from its use, he argued.

Then addressing the damages portion of my argument, Marion
argued that though their verdict should be for the Defense, he had a
duty to comment on Plaintiffs' argument on damages. Intentionally
keeping it very brief, he argued that if the jury did feel there was
liability on Ortho, a million dollars was "too much money" for this
case, and further that all the money in the world would not give
Michelle back her sight.

He closed by repeating to the jury it would be a hard decision
to turn Michelle away without a recovery by rendering a verdict
for the Defense, but justice, the evidence, and their oath required
them to do just that. Marion then thanked the ladies and gentlemen
of the jury for their time.

"Thank you, counsel. We will take a fifteen-minute recess, and
then counsel for Plaintiffs will give their closing argument," Judge
Allen said.

⁂

I became concerned about holding the jury much longer to hear a
lengthy rebuttal from me after sitting through seven weeks of trial,
but there was so much to rebut. A plaintiff's rebuttal argument

is limited by law to addressing *only* the subjects raised by the
defense in their summation. I was restricted from bringing up any
new evidence or issues not discussed in the defense argument.

◌∾

When we returned from the break, I began my final argument:
"Let me start with the initial question in this case that you
must answer with your verdict. Does the 'Pill' cause clotting in
some women? Mr. Pothoven just argued to you that it does not.
He is wrong. The evidence of causation which we presented over
these seven weeks of trial should appear to you as overwhelming.
An apropos quote from Hamlet cited in Dr. Schatz's article, in
evidence, reporting six challenge and response cases, says it all:
'Find out this cause of this effect, or rather, the cause of this defect,
for this effect defective comes from cause.'

"I think this sums up causation of the 'Pill.' A statement in the
conclusion of Dr. Schatz's article published in JAMA [The Journal
of the American Medical Association] in 1964, rings true as to the
responsibility of Ortho and Johnson & Johnson here:

'Nevertheless, when clinical experience that a
compound may cause unexpected complications,
even in a few patients, the inference that an
etiological association may exist *must be considered
until disproved.* This does not necessarily mean that
the uses of such medication should be interdicted. It
does imply that physicians involved in its use should
be made more fully aware of the possibility of such
complications in susceptible individuals. The risks

and advantage of prescribing the drug must then be
assessed by each physician after he has weighed the
indication for its uses and the needs of the individual
patient.'

"Mr. Pothoven argued to you that we are trying to take birth control
pills off the market. He contends that such would be a major
detriment to the world in preventing overpopulation, and it would
deny women the freedom to make their own choice as to birth
control methods. He has completely misstated and misinterpreted
our position. As you remember, I told you in opening statement
at the very beginning of this trial that the purpose of this trial is
not to take the 'Pill' off the market. We are not contesting that the
'Pill' works as an oral contraceptive. What we are saying is that
the warnings are not sufficient for women to have the *freedom of
choice to determine whether they want to take a risk or not.* In this
context, if there is substantial evidence of a risk, though it may not
be conclusive and the risk is one of possible death, or blindness, or
paralysis, or any serious injury or illness, where should the benefit
of doubt lie with a responsible company? That's the issue here—a
woman has a right to know what are the risks before taking the
'Pill' so that she can make her own choice as to whether to take
that risk. Michelle wasn't given that choice, and if she had been,
she told you she would never had taken the 'Pill.'

"Mr. Pothoven told you that their own studies were more
scientific and reliable because they are prospective studies—studies
that follow the patients forward. He distinguished this from the
British studies and other retrospective studies that demonstrated

a causal relationship by arguing that retrospective studies are not that scientifically reliable.

"A retrospective study gathers a study population who have either died from thrombosis or suffered morbidity and then looks backwards to what percentage were on the 'Pill.' He ignores Dr. Ley's testimony that the opposite is true. In the industry prospective studies, they never used controls—such as a population of participants not taking the 'Pill' to compare with those who are taking it. The retrospective studies performed by independent epidemiologist always used a control population and for that reason were much *more* reliable than that of the industry. It is only in a prospective study that there is such a thing as a loss to follow-up as we demonstrated to be common in Dr. Goldzierher's so called prospective studies performed for Ortho.

"Dr. Vessey, one of the main authors of the British retrospective studies in evidence, summed up the evidence in 1974 wherein he wrote:

> 'All of these investigations are, of course, subject to the well-known difficulties of the retrospective approach. Considered together, however, they provide compelling evidence that oral contraceptives are associated with venous thrombosis and pulmonary embolism and strongly suggest that this association is one of *cause and effect*. Other independent findings support this view. Trends in the official mortality statistics for venous thrombosis and pulmonary embolism for young women in the United Kingdom and the United States are compatible

with the increase in the use of oral contraceptives
and with the estimates of the risk associated with
them . . . Estrogens have been implicated as a cause
of thromboembolism, both venous and arterial,
when given to men with prostatic cancer. Oral
contraceptives increase the circulating levels of
certain blood coagulation factors and alter platelet
behavior . . . Distinctive vascular lesions have been
found in women dying from thromboembolism while
using oral contraceptives.'

"In the face of this hard evidence, Mr. Pothoven telling you vascular
lesions have nothing to do with it is nonsense. Dr. Altshuler
testified he found peculiar vascular lesions in women on the 'Pill.'

"You have seen that Ortho won't admit the greater susceptibility
to thrombosis in women with Type A, B, or AB blood, a genetic
susceptibility found in early studies, and the consequent greater
risk when on oral contraceptives as seen in recent studies in
evidence. As Dr. Bettman, Dr. Altshuler and other witnesses
testified, this is what made Michelle a sitting duck for thrombosis.
Ortho continues to ignore this science."

I directed the jury, again, to the overwhelming evidence of
causation between the "Pill" and thrombosis, despite the artificial
controversy created by the pharmaceutical manufacturers:

"Mr. Pothoven told you that Dr. Vessey and the many other
scientists who did the published studies had a vested interest in
attacking the 'Pill.' As you examine the source of the information,
you have to ask why is there a controversy, how did it get there,
why does it continue? Dr. Vessey is a British epidemiologist

employed by the British government. Where is his vested interest? In public health? I can certainly understand Dr. Goldzeirher having a vested interest. He was paid by Ortho to help get the 'Pill' on the market. Dr. Cronk certainly has a vested interest. He is the Medical Director of the Defendant in this case, Ortho. What can one expect him to say—our 'Pill' causes thrombosis and just didn't bother to tell anyone? I am not saying necessarily these people are dishonest, but what is naturally going to be their motivation? What bias subconsciously cause them to become convinced on key issues involving their company? Ortho, the company itself, has a bias. The evidence showed they had 28 percent of the 'Pill' market producing over 40 million dollars a year. How much motivation for bias does a company need? You must use your common sense in evaluating the evidence they produce verses ours.

"So, what did Ortho do wrong, Mr. Pothoven asked? They failed to test their product for its safety in a scientific manner; they failed to warn physicians and patients of known risks that came to their attention; they failed to alert them to current studies and adverse reports on their product; and they even went further misrepresenting what they did know."

I, again, addressed the question: Did Ortho-Novum cause Michelle's blindness? I pointed out the specific testimony of the treating doctors that confirmed the inability to isolate a source of infection in Michelle, and further, their own admissions that they did not know what caused her blindness. I further reminded the jury of the bias innately present in witnesses who did not believe the "Pill" caused clotting at all. I emphasized that not a single expert witness, Defense or Plaintiff, could point to a single case of bilateral blindness having been caused by a sore throat. I re-emphasized the power of logic contained in the challenge and response cases and, especially, the triple challenge and response case experienced by Dr. Harris, the very first witness in the case. I reminded them that these challenge and response cases are what finally convinced even the FDA Commissioner, that a *cause and effect* relationship truly existed.

I closed my final argument with the following quoted testimony from Michelle:

"Did anyone tell you that something like this could happen from being on the 'Pill'?"

"No."

"Were you ever given your choice of going on oral contraceptives and assuming the risk of blindness or death, or not going on the 'Pill'?"

"No, I wasn't."

I allowed my previous damage argument to stand with no further comment, ending:

"Ladies and gentlemen, I hope your verdict will be a meaningful verdict in answering the questions presented to you in this case. I thank you for your time and diligence during this long trial."

෭෨

Judge Allen then gave the jury a fifteen-minute recess after which he instructed the jury on the law applicable to the case. He gave them the special verdict form which contained a special question to be answered with their verdict: "Was Ortho-Novum a substantial factor in bringing about Michelle Ahearn's blindness. Yes_____ No_____."

At 3:55 p.m. on Thursday, December 12, 1974, the Court sent the jury to the jury room instructing them to select a foreperson who would lead their deliberations on the case and then report back to the courtroom to be dismissed for the day.

Upon entering the jury room, a juror suggested they all hold hands and pray before doing anything on the case and they did so. They then proceeded to nominate and select their foreperson to lead the jury. They chose one of the most highly educated among them, a pleasant professional woman in her mid-fifties. She was the juror with two master's degrees, one in psychology, and an extensive background in epidemiology. She was the prolific reader of professional and scientific literature.

They then knocked on the jury room door which called the bailiff, at which time they told him they were ready to return to the courtroom. The foreperson, now the spokesperson for the jury, advised the Court they had completed their task. At 4:28 p.m. that afternoon Judge Allen dismissed them for the day to allow them to return fresh the next morning to start deliberations.

രൂ

As the jury walked out of the courtroom, Harold and I, standing in the required respectful manner to the jury, whispered to one another, "What a great choice for a foreperson for this case," and then followed them out, picking up Michelle and Dennis along the way. Dennis stopped on the way out to converse with Marion.

When Dennis approached Marion he surprisingly said, "Mr. Pothoven, do you know what I don't like about you?"

Marion, not knowing what to anticipate, replied, "What?"

"You're too good," Dennis said and walked away.

We then all continued walking out of the courthouse together away from the jury, I explained to Michelle and Dennis that we were pleased with the jury choice of a foreperson. Her questions to various witnesses during the trial demonstrated she clearly understood the medical and legal issues that most concerned us.

"So far, so good," I commented.

We were somewhat relieved that the battle was over and resigned to the fact that the case was now in the hands of the jury. There was nothing more we could do to affect their judgment on the case. I asked Michelle and Dennis their thoughts on how summation went. Michelle, replied without hesitation, "I think you nailed it, Sal. You went point by point on all the testimony that proved what Ortho was doing. In my mind, how can any reasonable person not come back with a verdict for us? I don't see how they could ignore what the company did?"

Of course, I was appreciative of the compliment, but well experienced with the unpredictability of jurors. I was concerned that Michelle and Dennis were too confident of a win. Yet, considering what they had been through, I didn't want to take away their momentary positive feelings.

Dennis added, "The Defense never came back to refute— Pothoven didn't have any way to dispute that stuff."

"I hope you're both right, and the jury saw it that way," I countered. "But we will soon find out." I asked if they were comfortable with my asking the jury for over a million dollars?

Dennis commented, "The president of Johnson & Johnson made over $1 million in a single year."

Although this was true, it was not proper to introduce into evidence since the Court ruled earlier we would not be allowed to seek punitive damages in this case.

∽

We got back together for dinner that evening at a local restaurant to reminisce many parts of the case, especially now that the pressure of facing another day of trial was off. Harold and I were joined by his wife, Betty; my wife, Laura; my paralegal, Betty; and my dad, Sam. Betty and my dad observed most of the trial and were great contributors to evaluating the day by day progress, especially their observation of the jury's reaction to particular evidence as it came in. The location of their seats in the audience of the courtroom provided a clear vision of each of the jurors and would often provide helpful insight on their individual reactions.

That evening I felt better about our chances of winning as did Harold, but we both knew anything can happen in the jury room to result in a loss. I retired exhausted but enthused that my clients truly felt they were not only vindicated in their willingness to go to trial on this unpopular case, but truly convinced from the evidence they heard at trial that they did the right thing. They felt thoroughly vindicated in proceeding with this lawsuit, despite their basic anti-litigation philosophy. Michelle repeated several times her belief that this case would save many other women from going through what she suffered, and to her, that made the entire effort and risk worthwhile.

CHAPTER 12
The Verdict

We returned to the courtroom the next morning to be present during deliberations and, particularly, in case the jury sent notes to the judge with specific questions. More importantly, the jury could reach a verdict at any time. True jury deliberation on the issues of the case began in earnest on that Friday, December 13th, at 9:05 a.m. (Yes, a Friday the 13th).

During deliberations that day, the jury returned to the courtroom with questions requesting clarification or further instructions from the Court on four different occasions. Typically, as trial lawyers we strain to read some meaning out of their questions as to where they are in their deliberations. The questions later in the day seemed to concern their tasks of addressing damage issues in the case, which somewhat relieved us, but not entirely. I had been fooled by that misinterpretation in the past. Harold and I both realized it was unlikely that the jury would have resolved such complicated liability issues in only a half a day of deliberations.

Shortly following the jury inquiry that appeared to deal solely with damage issues, Marion approached me with a very unexpected question.

"What amount of money will it take to settle this case?"

Prior to the commencement of trial, we had offered to settle the entire case for both Michelle and Dennis for one million dollars. The only response from Ortho up to that time was a grand total of $75,000. The costs I had already incurred to prepare and try the case to that point exceeded their offer. If we had accepted, there would have been nothing left for Michelle and Dennis.

Ortho up to that time, had been quite confident they would get a Defense verdict thereby winning the case. If they were to succeed, they could then come after Michelle and Dennis for a large part of their out of pocket costs which most probably exceeded mine. Ortho had spent a lot of money in fighting this case. That potential reality added a lot of stress to Michelle and Dennis in any settlement negotiations. They were far from being a wealthy family. Contrarily, they were financially struggling, especially at this point of time having to spend substantial money to accommodate Michelle's living with her blindness and all the financial consequences that flowed therefrom. Having been so far apart in our negotiations in the past, I did not expect Johnson & Johnson to be interested in any settlement amount in the seven-figure range now that the case had been tried and was in the hands of the jury.

I approached Michelle and Dennis, who were with me in the courtroom the entire time during jury deliberation and relayed the message from the Defense.

"What do you think are our chances of winning?" they asked.

"I feel the trial went very well, but one can never predict with certainty what any jury will do. It is always unpredictable until the verdict is entered into the record. It would not be right for me to gamble with your money by telling you not to negotiate. That has to be your decision."

"Okay," Dennis responded, "What do you need from us?"

"What amount of money would satisfy you at this juncture— leave you with the feeling that you had received justice?" I responded.

They stepped away and discussed it between themselves for a few moments, before returning to me with their offer.

"We've made a decision," Dennis stated. "Tell them we will settle for $750,000. That seems adequate and fair to us."

They were, no doubt, motivated to bringing an end to the stress surrounding the risk of total loss. I felt they made the right decision and immediately passed that offer onto Marion to communicate to his client. I told Marion that having already incurred the expense of the trial, that was not an unfair amount to be demanding.

Michelle and Dennis had not previously been interested in any compromised settlement knowing that if such occurred prior to trial, it would be conditioned upon the entire case being sealed under a confidentiality order. A major motive for their going through trial was to educate the world on the dangers of the "Pill" which would save many lives and prevent even more from suffering the human misery from thrombosis consequences. At this point, that goal had pretty much been accomplished. Almost every trial day received extensive coverage by the local press and often in other major cities within the U.S. The American medical profession and women had now been exposed to the truth nationwide.

When I passed this offer onto Marion, he surprisingly stated, "Their offer is fair at this stage of the case, I will recommend it to my client."

I was surprised by Marion's response.

He shared with me he believed the amount was reasonable based upon how well the trial had gone for us and the serious nature of her injury. He explained that settlement offers for this case were controlled by the parent corporation, Johnson & Johnson's Chief Counsel, who happened to be a retired federal judge in the New York office.

c̓ℐᴏ

Marion insisted I stand next to him while he made the call to the judge so I could overhear the conversation. To be asked to listen in on such a conversation by a Defense lawyer was unheard of in my experience in the practice of personal injury law. I presumed his primary reason was there could be a knock on the jury door any second with an announcement from the bailiff that a verdict had been reached. So, he wanted me readily available in his conversation with the Chief Counsel to be able to quickly respond to any counter offers or questions.

Using a telephone booth located near our assigned courtroom, Marion made the call to the Chief Counsel's office in New York. Of course, neither of us knew what the status was of jury deliberations at that moment. I assumed that Marion's interpretation of the questions the jury was asking the Court was similar to mine indicating they had decided liability and were now deliberating on damages. We both knew a verdict could be reached at any moment. So, if a settlement was to be accomplished, time was of the essence.

As I stood next to Marion at the phone booth, I could clearly overhear his conversation with the Chief Counsel of Johnson & Johnson: "The Plaintiffs will take $750,000 to settle the case and I strongly recommend we pay it. The jury can reach a verdict any minute."

He received an immediate reply, "Tell them we will pay them $250,000 if they agree to settle now."

I was amazed that Johnson & Johnson would not take the advice of their own trial counsel. Who would be more informed on the jury's reaction to the evidence than the lawyer who tried the case? Yet, this retired federal judge sitting in his New York office of Johnson & Johnson, refused to listen to their own attorney.

Marion kept the judge on the phone while he asked me to quickly communicate the counteroffer to Michelle and Dennis. When I told them of the offer, Michelle's instant reaction was a very negative,"No way!" Dennis instantaneously agreed. I ran back to the phone booth and told Marion of their refusal. He again tried to get more authority, but Ortho's top claims person with authority to settle, this retired judge, would not give it to him. He slowly hung up the phone with a disturbed and disappointed look on his face. That was the last of any settlement discussions.

Jury deliberations continued until 4:28 p.m. that Friday the 13th, without reaching a verdict. The jury was released by Judge Allen and left the courtroom to reconvene on Monday, December 16th, at 9:15 a.m. to resume deliberations. As the jury filed out of the courthouse, Harold, Michelle, Dennis and I were standing outside chatting amongst ourselves and we glanced at their facial expressions looking for a "read." We were pleasantly surprised to see the jurors talking and smiling with each other in a very cordial manner. We interpreted this as a positive sign, although knowing it could be completely misleading as to what their mindset really was.

We began to anticipate that jury deliberations could go on for days. After all, the trial itself consumed 31 days, 3,840 pages of transcript, and 24 witnesses, including 18 medical doctors. Over 211 exhibits were marked for identification and most admitted into evidence, 115 having been offered by us Plaintiffs. For a jury to review and analyze all this evidence would certainly take several days.

On Monday morning, we returned to the courthouse prepared to spend the next several days waiting for a verdict. We watched the jury enter the jury room to continue deliberations. Shockingly to all of us, at 2:47 p.m. that Monday, the jury knocked on the door of the jury room and advised the bailiff they had reached a verdict. To us, that was too soon, and the fear of a Defense verdict raised its ugly head. The Court advised all parties to reassemble in the courtroom to receive the verdict.

The bailiff opened the door to the jury room and one by one each juror entered the courtroom taking their respective chairs in the jury box. Harold and I strained, looking into their faces searching for clues of their verdict. Usually, if they possess a serious, sad, even tearful look, with heads drooped toward the floor to ignore eye contact with the plaintiffs, the verdict most likely is for the Defense. Contrarily, if the verdict is in favor of the plaintiff, their faces would usually reflect a relaxed, sometimes even joyful look with smiles and eye contact with the plaintiffs.

As we stared, we immediately felt it was probably good news— at least on the issue of liability. They looked at Michelle and

Dennis with smiles and happy facial expressions. The question that immediately ran through both Harold's and my mind was how much did they award in damages? In an earlier "Pill" case, Harold had received a verdict for the plaintiff on liability, but damages were nominal, in the area of $20,000, not even enough to pay the out of pocket costs of the lawsuit. Dennis also read the facial expressions of the jurors as good news, but we all held our breath waiting to hear the verdict read.

In the traditional custom, Judge Allen asked the jury foreperson to hand the signed verdict form to the Court Clerk who then handed it to Judge Allen to review. It was not unusual for a verdict form to be improperly completed and require the Judge to have the jury return to the jury room for further deliberations to resolve any discrepancy. We tried to read the judge's facial reactions as Judge Allen read the verdict to himself. I noticed an unusual concerned look on his face and became worried—did the jury do something wrong?

All of this seemed to take forever despite actually occurring rather quickly. When Judge Allen began to hand the verdict form back to the Court Clerk, I was relieved that at least the form was correctly answered and we would now hear the verdict. The Court then asked the clerk to read out loud the entire verdict form with the jurors' answers into the Court record:

"IN THE SUPERIOR COURT OF THE COUNTY OF SANTA CLARA, STATE OF CALIFORNIA, MICHELLE AHEARN AND DENNIS AHEARN, PLAINTIFFS

vs. JOHNSON & JOHNSON, INC., ORTHO
PHARMACEUTICAL CORPORATION, AND LUCKY
STORES, DEFENDANTS

SPECIAL VERDICT:

We the jury in the above entitled action, find the following
Special Verdict on the questions submitted to us:
Was Ortho-Novum a substantial factor in bringing about
Michelle Ahearn's blindness?
Answer: Yes.

GENERAL VERDICT:

We the jury find in favor of the Plaintiffs, Michelle Ahearn
and Dennis Ahearn and against the Defendants, Johnson
& Johnson, Inc., Ortho Pharmaceutical Corporation and
Lucky Stores, and award damages as follows: to Plaintiff,
Michelle Ahearn, $1,142,586 and to Plaintiff, Dennis
Ahearn, $105,668."[7]

I suddenly heaved a huge sigh of relief and turning toward Harold,
observed the same. I looked back at Michelle and Dennis. Michelle
broke into tears; Dennis was shedding a few tears as well.

Following standard procedure, the Court then asked if either
party wanted the jury individually polled. Marion stated, "We
request the jury be polled, your Honor." Thereafter, each juror was
asked, "Is this your verdict?" as to the *general* verdict form (that
portion of the verdict specifying the amount of the awards). The

7   This 1974 verdict, adjusted for inflation, would amount to $6,041,549 in 2019.

response from each individual juror, without hesitation, was a firm "Yes."

Then each juror was polled on the *special* verdict question, "Was Ortho-Novum a substantial factor in bringing about the Plaintiff Michelle Ahearn's blindness?" Eleven jurors again with no hesitation responded, "Yes." One male juror hesitated, then responded, "undecided." Since only nine favorable votes are necessary for a plaintiff to win in a civil case under California law, there was never a question of a win for the plaintiffs from this jury.

The jury then revealed they had done something very unusual at the time they reached their verdict in the jury room. They were so upset at Johnson & Johnson, they drafted a written message they requested be communicated to the Board of Directors of Johnson & Johnson. They asked Judge Allen if it could be read into the Court record on the case. He properly denied their request because their message would not constitute a part of the official verdict, and therefore could not be read into the record.

We later asked the jury if we could read it, which they welcomed. It read as follows:

> "In deciding in favor of the Plaintiff, Michelle Ahearn, and awarding damages against the defending drug company and pharmaceutical dispenser, we, as a jury, would like to qualify our decision as not absolving any other drug company, pharmacy, attending physicians, or federal or state drug regulating organizations from protecting the user's right to choose. Even if only one user in millions may be adversely affected by a drug and that adverse reaction is only partially known, or a

suspected predisposing factor but of a serious or fatal nature, the drug should be accompanied with an unmistakable warning in lay person language. If any literature as to its use is seen by the user or is a part of the prescribing physician's instructions then the suggested warning should not be nullified in any way by further comments or instructions either by the drug company, dispenser or prescriber.

Suggested form: 'Some adverse reaction reports indicate that with the use of this drug some people may be predisposed to or have serious or even fatal reactions such as . . .'"

❧

Judge Allen thanked the jurors for their service, advised them that they were now free to discuss the case with anyone they chose and dismissed them from the case. As they left the jury box, each juror approached Michelle and gave her a big hug as well as Dennis. To the jury, Michelle and Dennis were obviously their heroes for making known to the world, through the jury's verdict, that the "Pill" was a killer to many women. Harold and I invited the jurors to join us at my office that evening to celebrate this victory against *corporate greed*.

In the tradition of civility among trial lawyers who are fierce advocates on behalf of their respective clients, Marion approached me to congratulate me on the win, shaking my hand.

I said to him, "You are a powerful advocate for your client. You did a great job in defending this case."

As Harold and I walked out of the courthouse with Michelle and Dennis, I asked Michelle what her feelings were when she heard the verdict.

"I wanted to jump up and shout, but I didn't dare. It was bittersweet. I just sat there and it was like a burden was taken off of me. I actually thought to myself, thank you God, I knew they were to blame. Now, everybody will know. I felt vindicated in my decision. I felt like they were to blame, and we were vindicated that we did the right thing. People will now know, in fact, what caused it and that I wasn't just suing for money."

Dennis followed with his thoughts, "Obviously, the money was secondary. The money aspect definitely has some value in that it will give us the resources to better deal with Michelle's blindness. But most important, was that what you proved was *true*. We had feelings from friends and others who thought we were just out to try to get money."

I invited them both to come to my office that evening to greet each of the jurors. I was fearful in all the immediate excitement they might overlook the importance of being there. Michele indicated they definitely would attend and looked forward to finally having the opportunity to talk with each of the jurors. Then Michelle said to me, "You know, Sal, I am your million-dollar baby!"

By evening, the *San Jose News* had already published the verdict in its front page headline article with Michelle and Dennis's photo.

Every juror attended our *Ahearn* victory party that evening. It was truly a grand celebration for everyone with wine and champagne flowing. Many jurors expressed feelings of pride that they had fulfilled an important public service that would not only bring justice for Michelle and Dennis, but at the same time would change the world for the better.

During our discussions with the jurors that evening, we learned that a favorable verdict was never in doubt. On the first vote within the first hour of deliberations on that Friday the 13th, they took up the special question on the verdict form as to whether the "Pill" caused Michelle's blindness. That first vote was 9 to 3 in favor of causation. That vote in itself was a sufficient number under the law to resolve that question favorable to Michelle. However, they explained that jurors wanted to continue to deliberate on liability and causation reaching a 10 to 2 vote shortly thereafter. Despite that number being more than adequate, they were striving for a unanimous 12 to 0 on liability. When they reached 11 to 1 they stopped. The single dissenter stated to the rest of the jurors that on the Special Verdict Form, he could not decide *one way or the other*, so that became the final vote on liability and causation. Having found that little time was necessary for them to decide liability, they proceeded to the *issue of damages*. At the beginning of that discussion they were very far apart from one another. However, through compromise over the next two days, they reached a consensus on the amount of damages for Michelle for her blindness, and for Dennis for his loss of consortium. [8]

⁓

For Harold and me, it was a big relief and accomplishment to have finally succeeded in a court of law against Big Pharma for distributing, without adequate warnings, a drug responsible for the death and morbidity of thousands of women—all for profit. After

---

8   The law allows a spouse to recover from the loss of love, companionship, services, etc. of an injured spouse referred to as consortium.

so many "Pill" cases being lost around the country, this appeared to finally be a turning point in the nationwide litigation.

The following day the verdict became headline news again in the morning newspaper, the *San Jose Mercury*.

BIRTH CONTROL PILL VICTIM—BLIND WINS FORTUNE

News also quickly spread throughout the nation, appearing in the *Chicago Tribune*, *New York Times*, the *Wall Street Journal*, and even newspapers around the world as far as Australia. Even Johnson & Johnson investors got the message—Johnson & Johnson's stock dropped five points that morning on the New York Stock Exchange.

༅

However, the local medical profession, particularly OB-GYNs, were very unhappy with the verdict. Two local OB-GYNs gave the press an extensive interview appearing on their plan to encourage OB-GYNs to no longer prescribe the "Pill" because the case put them all at risk of malpractice lawsuits, wrongfully assuming the *Ahearn* case was against the prescribing physician, rather than solely the pharmaceutical manufacturers and distributors. They failed to grasp that the verdict benefitted prescribing physicians, requiring that they as well as their patients be fully informed by Big Pharma. We had defended the doctors contending their lack of knowledge was solely the fault of the pharmaceutical industry, but they failed to get that message. These two local doctors were entirely ignorant of what the real issues were in this case and operated upon their own false assumptions, never inquiring as to what were the true facts.

Their scathing interview appeared on January 5, 1975 in the *San Jose Mercury*. They attacked the jurors' character personally, as being an emotional and *uneducated jury*. That could not have been further from the truth. The doctors also attacked Harold and me personally, as dishonest lawyers persuading jurors with emotional arguments to reach a false and dishonest verdict.

The doctors argued the "Pill" was safe and thoroughly tested. This again clearly demonstrated the thorough job the pharmaceutical manufacturers had done up to that time brainwashing physicians. They literally did not have a clue as to the catastrophic risks of the "Pill" and the amount of condemning evidence.

I replied to the article and the doctors themselves with a scathing critique of their quoted statements, demanding a retraction. I mailed it directly to their offices with a copy to the *San Jose Mercury* hoping it would be printed, but it was not.

✑

Several days following the verdict I met with Michelle and Dennis to advise them on what to expect from here. To them, the jury decided the case.

"Isn't it over?" they asked.

"Unfortunately, no."

I explained that typically in any case where there is a large verdict, you have to anticipate the defendants will make a motion before the trial court requesting a new trial on various legal grounds.

"This was an historical verdict for many reasons," I pointed out. "First of all, the industry can't afford to let it stand without a fight to reverse it. The verdict, itself, puts at risk for Big Pharma, every future trial in the hundreds if not thousands of pending cases around the country, and encourages the filing of many new cases. The verdict has the effect of educating trial lawyers around the country of the potential value of "Pill" cases, and the liability exposure of the industry.

"Secondly, the mere amount of this verdict is historical for the time. It is one of only a couple of dozen verdicts over a million dollars in the entire country, so Johnson & Johnson will try to do everything it can to convince the judge that it should be taken away or at least reduced."

"Does a judge have that power?" Michelle and Dennis both asked.

"Sadly, yes," I responded. "Last, but not least, if this verdict is allowed to stand, it will cost Johnson & Johnson millions of dollars in lost profits by a reduction in sales of the 'Pill.'"

"For the foregoing reasons," I explained, "a motion will probably be filed by the Defendants within the fifteen-day time period allowed under California Law," which was due to expire in a few days.

"It's rare that a trial judge will take away a verdict where the verdict itself was unanimous and the trial evidence was as favorable to the verdict as occurred here. I'm not worried the judge will tamper with the verdict in this case, nor should he."

Clearly frustrated, Dennis asked, "When does the case really come to an end?"

"The Defendants might take a shot at an appeal. The appellate court has the same power to reverse the verdict as the trial judge for insufficiency of the evidence to support the verdict, or even reduce the damages awarded by the jury if deemed too high. I don't anticipate this as a real problem in this case either, for the same reasons. If Johnson & Johnson lose in the Court of Appeals, they could petition the Supreme Court for a hearing, but it's not likely the Supreme Court would grant such a hearing in this case, for the same reasons."

These are among the many checks and balances against a non-meritorious or runaway verdict that our law provides.

✑

I informed them that many times a defendant will make an offer to settle *after* the verdict hoping to compromise the verdict amount in exchange for waving all their rights to appeal, and that was a real possibility in this case.

✑

Michelle and Dennis left my office with a better understanding of what procedures to anticipate but assured by me that there was a slim chance anything could change the verdict. They were prepared to anticipate a motion for a new trial by Johnson & Johnson.

CHAPTER 13
THE 13TH JUROR

The joy and happiness from the successful verdict still filled the hearts and minds of Michele, Dennis, the jurors, Harold and I, when Johnson & Johnson hit us with their timely Motion for a New Trial. *They filed on the very last day before the time limit to file ran out.* Although I anticipated their motion, it's always upsetting to the winning parties as well as their lawyers. However, I had hoped that having fought a long hard battle with such powerful evidence to convince a jury, almost unanimously, of the merits of our case, Johnson & Johnson would have raised the white flag and made the usual effort to settle for something a little below the verdict amount. I thought they would realize that a judge would not be anxious to take this verdict away, especially from a jury that was so articulate in its questions to the witnesses, as in this case. I was obviously wrong. To Johnson & Johnson, this was an historical loss that could destroy the marketability of their profitable product, the "Pill."

❦

The hearing date was set for January 30, 1975. Johnson & Johnson had ten days to file any affidavits and briefs in support of their motion, and we would have only ten days to respond with counter affidavits and our briefing on the issues they raised. This meant our work in this case was far from over before we could truly claim victory and success.

The major legal ground raised by Johnson & Johnson to support their motion was their claim that the evidence was insufficient to support the verdict rendered by the jury. This called into play the *13th juror—Judge Allen*. This issue raised by the Defense required us to retry the case on paper via written briefing and then oral argument before Judge Allen. No new or further evidence could be presented.

The judge is often referred to as the *13th juror* with the power to veto the twelve lay jurors. The most powerful influence of a judge is their ultimate interpretation of the evidence. If the judge disagrees with the jury's verdict, the judge has the power to take it away, under the law of California and most States. In other words, the judge must also weigh the evidence and ultimately reach a conclusion as to whether the verdict of the jury is supported by the evidence presented at trial. If the judge determines it is not, he or she has the power and the duty to reduce the amount of the verdict, or even reverse the entire verdict and order a new trial. The judge even has the power to go further and grant a verdict for the losing side.

Considering that now Judge Allen would be reweighing all the evidence, my fears increased as I reflected on his biased actions during the trial of the case compelling me to make a motion to recuse him for such bias. His initial comment at the beginning of the case in his chambers, when we described to him the nature of the case, came back to haunt me.

"I realize that if you made a study you would find a certain amount of people who are poisoned by table salt."

Knowing the significant role of scientific studies in our case, we had heard him discredit the evidentiary value of such studies before he had even heard the evidence. Now he alone would be deciding what values to put on those scientific studies and our experts who relied upon them. My fear continued to grow as these thoughts and memories wandered through my mind.

✑

The Defense gave their reasons. They claimed their experts supported the conclusion that strep alone was the *sole* cause of Michelle's blindness. Further, their witnesses testified that thrombosis could occur spontaneously in women without known cause. Their conclusion was that Michelle was just one of those unlucky people in which thrombosis occurs spontaneously. They claimed the Plaintiffs' expert witnesses did not have the qualifications to support their opinions, but only their experts were properly qualified.

The second statutory grounds cited in their motion was based on juror misconduct and irregularity of the proceedings. To support these specific grounds, the Defense filed three affidavits (declarations under oath). One affidavit was from one of the twelve jurors who decided the case in our favor. Johnson & Johnson obtained these affidavits by interviewing the juror either by phone or in person to obtain information they wanted to use in their motion. After the interview, the affidavits were prepared by the investigator or attorney—not by the jurors themselves. They managed to obtain the signature of one of the twelve jurors on the affidavit accusing two other jurors of improper conduct.

Mrs. Smith and Mrs. Brown were accused of discussing evidence from the case over lunch *during the trial* and relating such evidence to their own medical experiences. Specifically, Mr. Jones contended Mrs. Smith discussed experiencing certain side effects while on the "Pill" herself. This particular experience had already been disclosed to the Court and Counsel by Juror Smith during jury selection, yet the Defense accepted her as a juror at the time. Now, after the trial was over, they attacked that same juror as being biased against the "Pill." Mr. Jones' affidavit further contended that during deliberations Mrs. Smith "read to the other jurors a prepared statement about big corporations, how much money the drug companies were making, and they should be held responsible." His affidavit further accused Mrs. Brown, who became the foreperson of the jury, as unfairly conducting jury deliberations.

A second affidavit was filed by the Defense from an alternate juror, who did not participate in the deliberations, having never been placed on the jury, Mrs. White. Her affidavit accused juror, Mrs. Brown, of discussing the credibility of one of the Defense experts, Dr. McCabe, in the jury room in the presence of the entire jury and alternate jurors during the trial, and before deliberations.

While the trial was underway, the jury was requested by the Court to take breaks in the jury room to avoid contact with non-jurors who might attempt to communicate with them about the evidence in the case. So, the opportunity for jurors to have such discussions among themselves was certainly present, despite the repeated admonition from Judge Allen that they were not to discuss the case among themselves, or with anyone until they retired to deliberate at the end of trial.

A third affidavit was filed by Johnson & Johnson from one of their own attorneys, Mr. Varanini, accusing several jurors of improprieties among themselves based upon alleged statements to him by other jurors. This is "rank hearsay" in legal jargon. They further argued that the failure of one juror to respond to the special verdict question constituted irregularity in the proceeding under the law. This juror, when polled in the courtroom on the verdict form, stated that he could not say "yes" or "no" to the special verdict question of whether Ortho-Novum was a substantial factor in causing Michelle's blindness. The Defense argued that because this juror voted for the general verdict providing damages, that his vote was purely out of sympathy, and not based upon the evidence.

The affidavits, if true, presented a real concern and risk of reversal by Judge Allen. So, I rolled up my sleeves and went to work setting up appointments to personally visit and interview every single juror. I had my assistant, Betty, accompany me to be a witness to my interviews and record exactly what was said by each juror and alternate. My goal was to hopefully obtain sufficient counter affidavits to rebut what the Defense had filed.

I struck gold.

Not only was each and every juror and alternate receptive to my visit, but they were also very upset at being attacked when I related what the Defense had filed.

I was able to obtain thirteen counter affidavits completely and thoroughly contradicting what the Defense had filed. When interviewing Mr. Jones, whose affidavit was so heavily relied upon by the Defense in their briefing, he not only felt he had been misquoted in the affidavit about Mrs. Brown, and the others, but gave us a counter affidavit containing the following:

> "Each of the jurors including Mrs. Smith and Mrs. Brown made every effort and successfully avoided discussing or commenting upon any of the evidence during the course of trial and until such time as we were in deliberations. While in deliberations, Mrs. Brown was very fair in allowing each juror to express his or her reasons for their respective views and interpretations of the evidence. Mrs. Smith did not make reference to any particular knowledge or information contained in her background as to medical matters or anything else but relied entirely upon the evidence presented in this case."

As an interesting aside, when I interviewed the jurors, I asked what they thought about Judge Allen? Did they think he was fair to both sides? I inquired if they were influenced by the various comments Judge Allen had made throughout the trial, which in my view, favored the Defense contention of no causation between Ortho-Novum and Michelle's blindness. The response from all of them was that they thought Judge Allen was fair to both sides. They liked him and the way he ran the trial. They appreciated his allowing them to question witnesses themselves.

In the words of one juror, "Oh, we just thought that since the evidence was so overwhelmingly in favor of Michelle, he was just trying to level the playing field in fairness to the Defense."

That proved how wrong I was in my interpretation of the effect the Judge had on this jury. The jurors were clearly a lot smarter than even I had assumed. It also proved I made a huge mistake by making the motion for a mistrial. If it had been granted, I would have lost this excellent jury, since a new one would have to be picked. I, therefore, might never have obtained a Plaintiff verdict in this case.

✑

The third grounds for a new trial raised by Johnson & Johnson was that the "damages were excessive" and that I committed misconduct by asking the jurors in summation to put themselves in Michelle's shoes. This is referred to as a violation of the "golden rule." [9]

However, I had been misquoted by the Defense on the assertion that I violated the so called "golden rule." Their quote was not exactly what I had said based on the court reporter's transcript. Significantly, Judge Allen had overruled the Defense objection when I made that argument during summation, itself.

I could not believe that a trial judge would consider $1.2 million dollars excessive for bilateral permanent blindness. However, there were less than two dozen verdicts in the entire United States at that time that had even reached $1 million for a single plaintiff suffering personal injury or death. Further, there had never been a verdict that large against a pharmaceutical company for personal injury or death. So, the issue of excessive damages raised by Johnson & Johnson concerned me as well.

---

9   The "golden rule" argument asks the jurors to place themselves in the position of the plaintiff with regard to the injuries claimed in deciding the value of compensation, i.e., asking the jury what they would take for the loss of their vision?

The hearing for the Motion for New Trial was held six weeks after the verdict. Harold and I arrived at the courtroom with Michelle and Dennis. Except for the one subpoenaed juror, no other juror was present. Marion arrived with his assisting lawyer, Mr. Varanini. We cordially exchanged greetings. During the entire full day of argument and juror testimony, Judge Allen gave no clue as to how he might rule.

At the hearing the Defense subpoenaed into Court Juror Smith so that they could cross-examine her in an attempt to prove her bias against corporations, and specifically Johnson & Johnson. Mr. Varanini, who himself had signed the affidavit alleging she was biased, cross-examined her.

"The question would be whether or not this belief as to the corporate structure existed prior to the trial in this case or after the trial in this case."

She responded, "My husband has a corporation. It is a small one. Ford Motor Company is our parent company. It is a large corporation. I don't know very much about its structure . . . I don't bring any bias into the courtroom on the subject of corporations. That is all I can say. I do not come prepared to attack this company, and I went to great lengths to avoid doing just that."

༄

As to the assertion that she had made a prepared statement to the other jurors stating how much money drug companies were making, and that "they should be held responsible," she testified that no such statement ever existed. This fact of the non-existence of a prepared statement was restated in the counter affidavit of every other juror.

Judge Allen then took the matter under submission, meaning he would render his decision at a later time. Although this was typical, I was hoping he would not keep us in suspense.

✐

On February 7, 1975, Judge Allen filed his order.

He took away the verdict and granted a new trial to the Defense!

We were completely shocked by the judge's decision. He surprisingly exercised his power as the 13th juror with total veto power over the twelve lay jurors who almost unanimously had rendered a contrary verdict.

The order contained seven pages of reasons why he favored the Defense and was taking away the verdict of the jury. The grounds upon which Judge Allen granted a new trial were: (1) Irregularity in the proceedings, (2) Misconduct of the jury, (3) Excessive damages, and (4) Insufficiency of the evidence to support the verdict—each and every ground raised by the Defense. The Court relied upon all three affidavits filed by the Defense in its ruling on irregularity of the proceedings and misconduct of the jury. The thirteen counter affidavits from all twelve participating jurors and one alternate filed by us were completely discounted and ignored in Judge Allen's order. All of these had clearly denied the factual content of the three affidavits relied upon by the Court concerning the alleged jury misconduct. Yet, not one of our thirteen counter affidavits was ever considered or mentioned by the Court in seven pages of reasons in its Order.

Solely because the one juror was undecided as to the special verdict question on causation, the Trial Court concluded that the juror's decision on the general verdict awarding damages was "purely out of sympathy." That juror found against the Defendants on all other issues except that contained in the special verdict. Even though required by law, the judge gave no reasons, nor did he cite any evidence to support his conclusion. Further, as previously stated, the one vote of this particular juror was unnecessary to support the verdict since only nine votes are required under the law and we had eleven.

As further misconduct by the jury, the Trial Court cited the alleged conversation involving issues in the case by jurors while at lunch during trial. If such had occurred, it could have been deemed improper depending upon the particular issues discussed. In the jury affidavits we filed, all of the participating jurors denied such conversation ever occurred.

The Court further found the foreperson of the jury to be "an advocate for the Plaintiffs," and further to have concealed prior relevant experiences during voir dire questioning of the jurors at the beginning of the trial. This was simply not true and was strongly denied by the juror involved.

The Court relied upon the letter the jury composed to the Board of Directors of Johnson & Johnson as evidence of bias, even though it was written after they had reached their verdict. It represented opinion formulated by the jurors after they heard all the evidence in the case, which was certainly proper in my view. The judge also relied upon certain representations in the affidavit filed by Mr. Varanini, accusing certain jurors of misconduct based upon what other jurors told him. This was all hearsay and should not have been relied upon by the Court. Such misconduct was also denied by all twelve participating jurors in their individual affidavits. The judge pointed to certain questions asked of witnesses during trial, by a specific juror, as evidence of bias. However, he failed to cite anything specifically contained in the questions to support such a conclusion, as the law requires. Further, since nine other jurors who decided the case had not been criticized by the trial Judge in his order, the resultant verdict should have been left standing.

Yet, he took it away.

The Trial Court agreed the damages were "excessive" as well. Here again, he failed to specify in the entire seven pages of his order *why* he considered them excessive, as required by law. He did make general references to the "bias" of some jurors and a contention that my oral argument on damages at the end of trial was improper under the law as violating the "golden rule."

At the time I had made my argument, I referred to an amount of money that neither Michelle nor I would take for suffering blindness, if given such a choice. I did not make specific reference to what the jurors would take or not take for blindness. In other words, I did not ask the jurors to place themselves into Michelle's shoes in considering the amount of damages. The Court even misquoted the words I had used in his order. Further, the order ignored the fact that the Defense had objected at the time I was making the argument to the jury, yet Judge Allen immediately overruled the Defense. The implication of that ruling would be that my argument was proper.

He now appeared in his order to have changed his mind and ruling, but based upon an inaccurate recollection of what I had said. He obviously did not check the transcript, immediately available to him from the court reporter, to see what were the exact words I had used.

The next legal grounds upon which Judge Allen rested his order was "insufficiency of the evidence as to both the general and the special verdicts." He expressed his reasons:

> "The evidence is overwhelming that Plaintiff's blindness was caused by a severe infection of beta hemolytic streptococcus in the soft tissue of the throat, face, and blood stream and the oral contraceptive has no more connection with the loss of eyesight than Plaintiff's presence in California."

This conclusion of Judge Allen was, of course, contrary to the entire testimony of all of Plaintiffs' experts. Judge Allen went further stating that, "Every treating doctor reached this conclusion." This ignored the fact that three treating doctors who never themselves testified, Finkle, Noyes, and Brooks, indicated that thrombosis, and not infection alone, was the primary mechanism producing Michelle's blindness in their entries in the medical records. Their entries were testified to by both Plaintiff and Defense experts, and therefore constituted appropriate evidence for the jury to consider.

Further, contrary to the Judge's order, Dr. Kosmin testified that he could not explain the cause of blindness nor could the other treating doctors. Dr. Lippe testified, "I am not certain why Michelle is blind . . . I really cannot tell you exactly why Michelle went blind." However, he did not doubt that thrombosis was a major factor. Dr. Sogg had testified that venous obstruction (thrombosis) was a substantial factor in the overall problem. Last, but not least, none of the treating doctors even knew she was on the "Pill" at the time of her illness. The medical profession had never been told in the PDR or by Ortho's detail men of its risk in causing thrombosis.

As further justification for his order, Judge Allen contended that the "treating doctors' qualifications were unimpeachable." This statement ignores all the contrary evidence derived from their own testimony on cross-examination. He failed to even mention the extraordinary qualifications of the Plaintiffs' experts.

Judge Allen's order was that "the hospital records fully support the conclusion" that infection alone caused the blindness. As seen from the testimony, the hospital records were replete with evidence of thrombosis, and even reflected a working diagnosis of "cavernous sinus thrombosis." The records further confirmed the failure to locate a site of any infection other than the strep in the blood stream. Judge Allen added that, "Eminent independent experts who also testified for the Defense fully support the same conclusion." As we saw, witness after witness for the Defense on cross-examination provided strong proof of thrombosis as a cause, and not infection acting alone. The Judge further added to his reasons, "The only contrary evidence came from Plaintiffs' medical witnesses." This assertion ignored all the contrary evidence that came from the treating doctors and the Defense experts on cross-examination.

Finally, Judge Allen asserted that, "Plaintiff's medical witnesses were *less qualified*, never saw Plaintiff during her illness, and were not credible witnesses at this trial."

Just as the jury has the power to judge the credibility and qualifications of each witness, so does the trial judge. As the 13th juror with veto power over the twelve jurors, this became an overwhelming obstacle to deal with.

✍

As I sat in my office reading Judge Allen's order, which had just been received in the daily mail on the morning of February 10th, three days after it had been filed, I quickly came to the realization that we could well be at the losing end of this litigation, i.e., dead in the water. How do you convince an appellate court that the trial judge, who heard the evidence and observed the demeanor of the witnesses, is wrong in his judgment of who and what to believe and not believe?

I was sickened.

To be expected, Michelle and Dennis were devastated when I gave them the bad news. Michelle's immediate reaction was, "What the hell do we have a jury for?" She calmed down and added, "I think from his demeanor during trial, maybe he is biased in favor of the Defense from the standpoint that this is out of control—companies getting taken advantage of by these greedy lawyers."

Dennis was even more upset.

"This is unbelievable! Didn't he hear the same things we did? Didn't he hear the testimony and the truth? How could he do that? It was a unanimous decision of the jury. I remember during the trial that some of the time he looked like he was asleep or not paying attention."

When I called Harold to read him the order, he too was in disbelief and thoroughly upset.

The *San Jose News* front page headlines that afternoon, February 10, 1975, were brutal to read.

"$1.1 MILLION AWARD ERASED IN S.J. —JUDGE POINTS
OUT JURY MISCONDUCT"

"$1.1 MILLION JURY AWARD WIPED OUT."

The press even interviewed some of the jurors and dedicated an entire article to the subject the next day.

"TRIED THEIR BEST, SAY OVERRULED JURORS."

Among quotes from jurors, "I tried to the best of my ability. I still think it was a fair decision."

Another juror, "It's wrong to say we were biased or prejudiced."

A follow-up article appeared in the *San Jose Mercury* six days after Judge Allen's order, on February 13th, in which the very process upon which Judge Allen relied in part, i.e., obtaining affidavits from jurors disclosing details of their deliberation and prior mental beliefs, was brought into serious question and debate. The article was entitled: "RETRIAL BY AFFIDAVIT DRAWING FIRE." News of the Court's Order quickly spread across the United States

The day following the order, Johnson & Johnson's stock *rose* 5 points.

✑

I met with Michelle and Dennis to discuss the next step. They had three choices. They could completely drop the case at this point, if I could persuade Johnson & Johnson to waive their costs in exchange for our waiving an appeal. Second, they could appeal the Judge's Order. Third, they could choose to retry the case before another jury and possibly a new judge. I explained that our chance to reverse Judge Allen's decision was slim to impossible.

"It is up to you, Sal, but we want to go for an appeal," Michelle advised.

Dennis added, "We're shocked! Where do we go from here? This is a big miscarriage of justice, for crying out loud. How can a higher court let this stand? *Go for it!* We are completely right and the judge is wrong. What have we got to lose? I don't think there is any other course. If we stop here, they are just going to walk away from all the harm they have done."

As I read and reread Judge Allen's order over the subsequent days, a hidden nugget of gold began to emerge. His order did not mention whatsoever the other key issues in the case: Does Ortho-Novum cause blood clotting in some women at all? Does Ortho know that it causes blood clotting in some women? Should Ortho have known it caused blood clotting in some women? Did Ortho fail to warn on what they knew or should have known of these risks?

As a matter of law, the absence of any mention of the above issues would deem them resolved in Michelle's favor, if reviewed by an appellate court. In brief, we would not even have to address those issues on appeal, they would be deemed by the appellate court as supported by sufficient evidence in the judge's view.

If this appears strange, that's because it was.

CHAPTER 14
THREE JUSTICES WEIGH IN

My first inclination after reading Judge Allen's order was to quickly find an appellate specialist to assist me with an appeal. I had some appellate experience, but my initial reaction was this case would be too complicated for me to brief. To rebut the trial judge's reasons for taking away the verdict, the entire case would have to be retried in writing for the appellate court. Appellate courts do not hear testimony of witnesses. They rely solely upon the transcript of the testimony recorded at trial and briefing by both sides on the issues appealed.

I knew it was a rare situation where an appellate court would reverse a trial judge in this type of situation. Appellate Justices realize they are not in the position of the trial judge to physically observe the witnesses as they testify in order to determine credibility. I was fearful we were at the end of the road. Harold did not have the experience of appellate work that even I possessed, so he felt helpless in this situation as well.

I immediately researched the best appellate lawyers in California who handled plaintiff cases and sent them a copy of

Judge Allen's Order soliciting their help with an appeal. The responses were unanimous—they all refused. They all said the trial judge spent seven pages of his order spelling out his reasons. In their opinion that was all the law required. This was all he had to do for his order to be upheld on appeal. He is the 13th juror with veto power over the twelve lay jurors. The message could not have been clearer. They saw the case as a loser without a chance of success. None of these appellate lawyers, of course, had reviewed the transcript of the case and, therefore, did not know what the real evidence was. In my mind, in the entire seven pages of reasons stated in Judge Allen's order, not a single one was based upon the evidence at trial. Of course, only the lawyer who tried the case would know that.

There was one exception, a trial lawyer in Los Angeles with whom I was co-counsel in a Corvair trial against General Motors ten years earlier. David Harney was, to me, one of the most skilled, outstanding trial lawyers in America at the time, and equally skilled in appellate work with a history of great success. He was responsible for major product liability law advances in America during the 1960's, and considered an expert trial lawyer and writer in the field of medical malpractice. Although a lawyer only, his knowledge of medicine exceeded most doctors.

I sent Dave a copy of Judge Allen's Order asking for his help. He quickly responded urging me not to retain an appellate lawyer to appeal the case, but rather that I should handle the appeal myself. He pointed out that the trial was too factually complex for any lawyer but me to handle the appeal. He explained that to reverse Judge Allen I would have to literally retry the case on paper.

The procedure requires the losing party (Michelle), called the Appellant, to file the initial brief making the case for reversal of the trial judge's order. What Dave was saying to me, was that to reverse Judge Allen, I would have to present the most powerful evidence from the record of the trial, based upon my knowledge as the lawyer who tried the case. I had to convince at least two of the three Appellate Justices that the evidence in the case, cited from the transcript, was more than sufficient to support the jury's verdict. *And* that the trial judge's assertion of reasons was not supported by any evidence.

Since our experience with the Corvair litigation, I looked up to Dave as a mentor, not merely as a trial lawyer, especially in the field of product liability. In his early years as a lawyer he had been chosen to clerk for the Supreme Court of California which involved researching and drafting opinions for Supreme Court Justices. That gave him special insight as to the art of persuasion with appellate justices. Dave usually briefed and argued the appeals on the cases he, himself, had tried. I welcomed his advice and followed it, deciding to do the appeal myself. In reality, Dave had given me the only ray of hope I had received from anyone thus far.

About a week after receiving Dave's uplifting letter of advice, I received a letter out of the blue, from another great well-known trial lawyer whom I had never met, Melvin Belli. His letter was personal, as if we were friends. He told me he read in the "San Francisco Chronicle" how the judge had set aside my verdict, but he did not encourage me to appeal. Rather, he urged me, "Go after them again and get a bigger award next time." I assumed, he too considered an appeal hopeless, but rather I should waive an appeal and retry the case in accord with Judge Allen's Order.

The wisdom of Dave Harney was far more persuasive than all of the naysayers. The reality of the advantage I had in handling the appeal myself, as the lawyer who tried the case, was beginning to sink in. Unless the appellate lawyer had been present at the trial to observe the evidence, or had read and studied the transcript of the entire trial, that person would have no basis to know if the judge's stated reasons throughout the entire seven-page order were true or false. Clearly, I was the only person with this advantage.

∽

I began the long, rigorous journey of appealing Michelle's case, knowing success was against all odds. Coincidently, I saw an opportunity to attend a lecture by a great Supreme Court Justice, Matthew Tobriner, on how to write a brief that would encourage justices to read it, as well as be persuaded. One of his messages was that Appellate Justices spend only a few minutes reviewing a brief, so the brief must have a theme, just as any trial, and that theme has to be repeated throughout the brief. I took his advice and created the theme that in the entire seven pages of reasons contained within Judge Allen's Order, not a single reason was supported by the evidence. Without a doubt, his lecture could not have been more timely.

A rule of court limited appellate briefs to fifty pages. I could not envision how I could possibly present the evidence contained in over 3,800 pages of transcript to prove its "sufficiency" not only to uphold the verdict of the jury, but also that Judge Allen's Order was wrong—in only 50 pages. I applied to the Court of Appeals in San Francisco, to which this case had been assigned, for permission to double the page limit.

The Court granted my request, however I eventually discovered even that was not enough to retry this entire case on paper. Ultimately, my opening brief exceeded 130 pages, plus a huge appendix into which I dumped important testimony of witnesses, questions asked by the jurors, and other significant information crucial to demonstrating that Judge Allen was wrong.

My brief was filed on February 2, 1976—a full year of work.

✎

I felt I had done a good job in briefing the case, but my best encouragement came a few weeks later when I ran into a trial lawyer friend of mine in court on another case, Ned Good. He not only was a terrific trial lawyer, but also had a great reputation for his appellate work. Ned was on the Appellate Committee of the California Trial Lawyers Association (CTLA) whom I had asked to file an Amicus brief [10] before the Supreme Court of California, should I lose before the Court of Appeal. I therefore had provided CTLA with a copy of my opening brief, and Ned read it. He confided in me that once he started reading it, he couldn't put it down.
"It read like a novel and not a court brief," he said.

✎

The filing of my Opening Brief triggered the time deadline for the Defense to file their Brief in Opposition. I would then be required to file a Reply Brief, since as the Appellant, we again had the burden of proof. After all briefing had been completed, the Court of Appeals set a date for oral argument, a crucial procedure in this particular case.

---

10   A brief filed by a third party in support of one of the parties in the case as a "friend of the court."

Johnson & Johnson changed law firms for the appeal, hiring Bronson & Bronson, an elite San Francisco law firm, and particularly Edward Bronson, Jr., who had the reputation as an outstanding appellate defense lawyer. I had a lot of respect for Ed as a civil and ethical defense lawyer and we developed a friendly relationship during this case. At one point before the oral argument on the case, we had a serious discussion on the merits.

Ed, in a friendly but academic tone advised, "Sal, you don't really think you have a chance under the law to win this case, do you? The law is against you. The judge is the 13th juror with veto power over the entire jury."

"Ed, I agree that the odds are against me, but the Judge was wrong in his reasons. You didn't have the opportunity of experiencing the trial, itself, as I did."

✑

I appeared for oral argument in early January 1977, still convinced that I was in an uphill battle, and that the odds were strongly against seeing any success at the appellate level. Michelle, Dennis and Harold joined me at the hearing. I had advised all of them of my pessimism, yet Michelle, with her strong optimistic beliefs continued to exhibit her faith that we would somehow succeed because we were on the side of justice.

We alighted from the elevator on the third floor in this austere San Francisco building which housed the Appellate Courts and the Supreme Court of California. I searched the headings of the courtrooms until I found, "First Appellate District, Division One." As we entered, Michelle and Dennis were in awe of the majestic room. Although there were several lawyers sitting with their clients, an imposing silence filled the room. Soon, the Clerk of the Court announced for all to stand. The three appellate justices entered the room from a side door to the elevated platform where the bench was situated, below a large wood relief of the Great Seal of California. Justice Molinari was the Presiding Justice for that Court, sitting with Justices Elkington and Sims. The clerk then called the first case which was not ours.

The contrast to a trial court is quite astonishing. The lawyers for each side took their positions at the counsel table and the lawyer for the appellant then stood and approached the speaker's podium awaiting instructions from the Presiding Justice to proceed with argument. Argument itself is low keyed and academic in an appellate court, quite a contrast to the fiery arguments often seen in jury trials.

When our case was finally called, I stepped up to the podium and waited the signal from Justice Molinari to proceed. Addressing the Court, I first apologized for having exceeded the one hundred-page extended limitation for my opening brief, not knowing what to expect for such a rule violation. To my surprise and immediate relief, Justice Molinari responded, "Counsel, you need not apologize, it was an excellent brief." This was shocker number one for the day!

The second shock came seconds later as I began my opening argument. Justice Molinari interrupted me in the middle of my very first sentence.

"Counsel, unless you insist, we would rather hear from the Respondent at this time."

I immediately replied I would reserve my time and I sat down. I wondered with that comment, had the case done a 180-degree reversal and was now running in our favor?

Justice Molinari then did the same to Ed Bronson—interrupting his very first sentence with a question.

"Counsel, before you go any further, we would appreciate your addressing one question we have. Can you point out to us from anywhere within Judge Allen's seven pages of reasons, one reason that is supported by the evidence that exists within the entire transcript of the trial?"

This was the theme of my briefing, that not a single reason stated by Judge Allen in his Order was supported by any evidence in the entire transcript of the trial.

Ed tried his best as a skilled appellate lawyer to rationalize an answer for the Court, but it became evident to everyone he was not persuasive that any such supportive evidence existed.

Observing the Court's continued questioning of Ed, it appeared clear to me that we were over the hill on the major issue of insufficiency of the evidence to support the jury verdict, and even further, that the Court was not impressed with any of the other grounds cited by Judge Allen to justify taking away the verdict, or even reducing it.

After Ed had exhausted his allowed time, I responded with only a brief summary of our position, knowing the Court had read and digested my briefing in the case.

∽

With a sigh of relief, I joined Harold, Michelle, and Dennis and walked out of that Appellate courtroom realizing for the first time in over a year that we had a decent chance to restore the jury's verdict. Harold, breathing a huge sigh of relief as well, explained to Michelle and Dennis what had occurred.

I added, "Based upon the Court's questioning, the odds are now clearly in our favor. It is highly unusual in my appellate experience to have the court signal its position so clearly on the issues of a case during oral argument, as we just witnessed."

As Michelle and Dennis began to relax, Ed Bronson approached me.

"You did a great job. It isn't looking too good for me."

∽

On March 16, 1977, the Court of Appeal filed its fifty-page opinion containing its decision in the case. The opinion was written by Justice Elkington but was unanimously signed by all three Justices.[11]

The opinion began: "Our principal inquiry is whether there was 'substantial basis in the record' for the 'reasons' given by the trial court in granting Defendants a new trial in the instant case."

Here, the Court relied upon the law that required there be a "substantial basis in the record" for the reasons stated by the Trial Judge.[12] They did a thorough analysis of the substantial evidence presented at trial as contained in the transcript.

Thereafter, they analyzed Judge Allen's Order point by point:

> "But the principal factual issue of the trial was
> whether Ortho-Novum had a tendency to cause

---

11   Appellate Opinion in its entirety can be obtained from the author.
12   California Code of Civil Procedure, Section 657

thrombosis in its users. The court's 'reasons' did not indicate its resolution of that issue. A lesser, but nevertheless important, issue was that assuming such a thrombosis-causing tendency of Ortho-Novum did it, in Michelle's case, cause the thrombosis and blindness? Again, the court's 'reasons' give no indication of its conclusion, from the evidence, on that issue. The 'reasons' were not 'sufficiently precise to permit meaningful appellate review,' for we are given no information how the court evaluated the evidence on each of those major issues."

The Appellate opinion then pointed out that Judge Allen made no mention of his reasons, based upon the evidence, on several key issues.

"It is, therefore, for our purposes, established (1) that Ortho-Novum does tend to cause blood clotting, (2) that Ortho knew of this tendency and did not give reasonable notice thereof, and (3) that Michelle had no knowledge of Ortho-Novum's blood clotting tendency, and would not have used the product had she known."

It thus appeared to the Appellate Justices that Judge Allen did not dispute that the "Pill" caused blood clotting in some women in his order, or that Ortho's warnings were adequate, but he only contended infection alone, and not the "Pill" was the only cause of Michelle's blindness.

Narrowing in on that logical interpretation of Judge Allen's Order, the Appellate Justices further stated:

> "We find it to be an established fact of the case that thrombosis, from some cause, proximately and substantially contributed to Michelle's blindness; the record offers no reasonable basis for a finding to the contrary . . . The testimony of defendants' medical experts standing alone, or added to that of the three 'treating doctors' must also be said to furnish no 'substantial basis' for the trial court's 'reasons' presently under consideration. . . Accordingly, no 'substantial basis is found in the record' for the trial court's stated reasons for granting a new trial on the ground (of) . . . Insufficiency of the evidence to justify both general and the special verdicts."

The Justices then reviewed the trial court's reasons for reversing upon "excessive damages."

> "'It is mandatory and jurisdictional'" that sufficient reasons be stated in support of an order granting a new trial on the ground of 'excessive damages.' In their absence, as here, the order becomes invalid on that ground, as to which ground 'the judgment will be automatically reinstated . . .'"

They addressed the remaining grounds used by the trial court to take away the verdict, *Irregularity of the Proceedings*, and *Misconduct of the Jury*.

"Our consideration of the foregoing 'reasons' given by the trial court in support of a new trial on grounds of misconduct and irregularity, of the jury impels us to declare as a matter of law, that they singly and collectively furnish no reasonable or 'substantial basis' for a new trial on those grounds."

The justices likewise held the trial court's quote of my so-called violation of the "golden rule" in my summation to the jury was erroneous. After reviewing that portion of my summation from the transcript, they found no misconduct or error.

Finally, this Court of Appeal stated its decision in the case, "*The order granting a new trial is reversed and the judgment is affirmed. Plaintiff to recover their cost of appeal.*"

We won!

But with a caveat.

The Court of Appeals Opinion was stamped in large letters at the top:

"NOT TO BE PUBLISHED IN OFFICIAL REPORTS."

That meant this case could not be cited as precedence in any court of law in any other case. Appellate courts have such discretion whenever they file an Opinion on a case. The reasons are not always so clear. Our guess in this case was the Opinion was critical of the lower court's order—but we will never really know for sure.

I immediately called Harold and told him the good news. He, of course, was ecstatic. I could not reach Michelle and Dennis because they were visiting a relative in Orange County but heard the result through the local media. Michelle described how she and Dennis were yelling, shouting and hollering, "We won! We won! We can't believe it."

"Thank you, God," she said. "Maybe there is justice after all."

"Well, Honey, I guess I'm married to a millionaire again." Dennis exclaimed. The headlines announced the reversal on March 19, 1977.

"EARLIER VERDICT REVERSED—$1.1 MILLION FOR BLIND WOMAN"

The reversal was again picked up by the press around the world. And again Johnson & Johnson stock *dropped* five points on the stock market.

The question in my mind at that moment, "Is this really the end to this historic journey that began way back in 1969?" Unfortunately, the answer was, no. Johnson & Johnson shortly thereafter filed a Petition for Rehearing on April 1,1977, before the same Court of Appeals in a last ditch attempt to persuade the Court to reverse their decision. This required more responsive briefing by us. Fortunately, two weeks later, on April 15, 1977, the Appellate Court denied their petition. We had filed a request to the Court to publish the opinion, so it could be cited in later cases as authority, but that was also denied at the same time.

Following that denial, as expected, Johnson & Johnson filed a Petition for Hearing before the Supreme Court of California.

CHAPTER 15
THE CALIFORNIA SUPREME COURT—
THE FINAL ANSWER

An appeal to the Supreme Court of California is in the form of a Petition for Hearing, which is rarely granted. It requires the vote of at least four of the seven justices on the Court. The Court reviews the original briefs of the parties filed in the Court of Appeal, along with the Court of Appeal's written opinion. A hearing will only be granted when four of the seven Supreme Court justices disagree with the Court of Appeal, and when the legal issues are critical to the advancement of the law, and/or that the lower court opinions are in conflict.

༄

I called Michelle and Dennis to inform them, as anticipated, Johnson & Johnson was petitioning the Supreme Court of California. Dennis answered the phone and immediately exclaimed, "Here we go again! We have been reinforced by the Court of Appeal decision on the verdict. What could the Supreme Court see that they would reverse the Court of Appeals?"

Michelle on the other line added, "If three justices found sufficient reason to reverse Judge Allen, I honestly feel we have a terrific chance. There is a certain amount of Providence in this."

"The odds are on our side this time," Dennis said.

I replied, "I generally agree with you, but as you know, there is no guarantee of success."

Knowing the impact of the *Ahearn* case on society, and its notoriety in the press, we were fearful they would grant a hearing. If so, there was always the chance the Defense briefs could influence the Court to reverse the Court of Appeals and sustain Judge Allen's Order granting a new trial. We waited on pins and needles with growing suspense to learn what the initial ruling would be—would they grant or deny a hearing?

With a six-man and one-woman Court, I had reason to be concerned. However, I had the privilege of personally knowing and working with the Chief Justice of the Supreme Court, Rose Bird, years earlier when she was the Public Defender of Santa Clara County. Justice Bird was appointed by Governor Jerry Brown during his first term as Governor of the State of California and was the only woman on the Supreme Court. She was also the first female Chief Justice to have ever been appointed to the Court.

When Justice Bird was a practicing lawyer and the Public Defender, we were both on the Board of the Santa Clara County Bar Association. I then had the opportunity to work together with her on several legal projects important to the County Bar and the public. I experienced first-hand her intelligent, yet pragmatic approach to problem solving issues within the law. She was not only ethical and competent as an attorney, but very knowledgeable.

I found her judicial opinions as Chief Justice on the Court to be well reasoned and yet courageous when dealing with unpopular subjects. For those reasons, I consequently felt somewhat confident that she would understand the serious complex issues involved in Michelle's case, particularly in that the case was truly a woman's cause.

In the late morning hours of June 23, 1977, I received an unusual call from the Clerk of the Supreme Court. I did not know him personally, so I was somewhat concerned when my secretary told me who was on the phone. He asked if I was Mr. Liccardo?

"Yes," I answered.

He informed me that the Supreme Court had reached a decision in the *Ahearn* case denying a hearing.

We had won—again!

The usual procedure would have been to receive a written ruling from the Court a day or two following their decision, so I was surprised by the call. I immediately called Michelle and Dennis to share the good news—they were ecstatic. I informed Harold and then my office, all of whom were overjoyed and relieved.

It was finally over.

⟋⟍

The next day I received the written decision, a simple postcard stating "Hearing denied." Two Supreme Court Justices, William Clark and Frank Richardson voted against us in favor of granting the petition for a hearing. Four justices voted in our favor: Chief Justice Rose Bird, Mathew Tobriner, Wiley Manuel, and Stanley

Mosk.[13] Their opposition to granting a hearing automatically reinstated the lower Court of Appeal's decision as the law of the case, thereby bringing the litigation to a final end.

By this action, the verdict was then reinstated for the last time.

With this decision by the California Supreme Court, Johnson & Johnson had nowhere else to go. Ordinarily the last step after a decision from the state's highest court would be to Petition the Supreme Court of the United States, but there being no Federal issue involved in the case, there was no legal basis to do so.

The long eight-year battle *finally* came to an end—David won; Goliath lost!

The June 24, 1977, *San Jose Mercury* headlines read:

"WOMAN BLINDED BY THE PILL TO KEEP $1.1 MILLION AWARD."

The article retraced the entire litigation's ups and downs to this ultimate conclusion of a final win. Other newspapers from around the world spread the good news. The litigation was *FINALLY* over.

✑

Johnson & Johnson's counsel, Ed Bronson, Jr. called me that day, "Congratulations, Sal. My client said they will immediately pay the judgment if your clients will waive the interest."

Almost three years had passed since the original judgment had been entered, so the legal rate of seven percent interest on a judgment of $1.2 million dollars had added up to a significant sum by that time, over $200,000. Knowing that Johnson & Johnson had no legal basis to continue the litigation to any higher court, I replied to Ed.

---

13   Coincidentally it was Justice Tobriner's lecture that assisted me in drafting my brief to the Court of Appeal.

"As you know, Ed, there's no place else for Johnson & Johnson to go, so I can't possibly recommend this to my clients, to compromise that much. Knowing my clients, I'm sure they wouldn't accept that in any event. They have nothing to gain."

Ed courteously replied, "I assumed that much and I'm merely carrying out my client's request. I'll ask them to issue a draft as soon as possible with full interest."

Johnson & Johnson thereafter timely paid every penny of the judgment, cost of appeal, plus the interest from the date it was entered on December 1974.

I anticipated that Johnson & Johnson stock would again drop five points on the New York Stock Exchange once it reached the press. Sure enough, the next morning the stock again dropped five points. That drop gave me great satisfaction to know they were paying, even with the value of their stock, for the fraud they committed on American women.

✐

Of equal benefit to our system of trial by jury, was the Supreme Court's vindication of our jurors. In rendering their verdict against a major oral contraceptive manufacturer, they demonstrated tremendous courage in their willingness to challenge public opinion, as well as the current beliefs of the entire medical world. These particular jurors gave up seven weeks of their life to perform their duty as jurors in a very complex and difficult case. Their compensation in dollars was a token amount. To follow and understand the scientific and medical evidence required serious, conscientious mental work for each of them. For some of the women jurors who were either on the "Pill" or had been on it at some time, this case required them to question the safety of a prescriptive drug recommended by their own personal physician.

Judge Allen had told these jurors at the beginning of trial that one compensation for being a juror in this case was that they would learn a lot of medicine. And that they did!

The dedication and desire to work hard to come up with the truth was evidenced by the many technical, intelligent questions they themselves asked each witness orally at the end of each examination. I had incorporated most of their questions in my opening brief to the Court of Appeals to illustrate that this was a jury not swayed by emotion, but by logic and intelligence. There is no doubt in my mind that the Court of Appeals and the Supreme Court were impressed after reviewing those jurors' questions.

After such diligent work and real sacrifice on the part of these jurors, to have the Trial Judge wipe out their end product with one sweep of the pen, and then accuse them of *bias* was more than shocking and disappointing; it was a serious blow to their confidence in the system of justice. Then to be accused of *jury misconduct* added insult to injury. Judge Allen delivered a final blow when he ruled the evidence they had worked so hard to understand and scrutinize was *insufficient evidence* upon which to reach their verdict.

As if this attack on their personal integrity was not enough, they then suffered the humiliation and embarrassment of seeing front-page coverage in their own hometown newspaper of Judge Allen's criticism of their verdict and their personal conduct, some jurors even being expressly named. They further faced open criticism from certain medical doctors eager to be quoted in the press on their opinion that the jurors were incompetent and too uneducated to decide this case. They claimed the jurors were motivated solely by emotional sympathy for the Plaintiff, Michelle. To say that many, if not all of the jurors, felt their contribution of their valuable time to our system of justice was completely wasted—would be an understatement.

Fortunately, two years after Judge Allen's Order, the jurors were completely vindicated by three appellate justices who not only reasoned that the jury did *not* commit any misconduct under the law, but further had based their verdict on overwhelmingly *sufficient evidence* to support it.

A majority of the Supreme Court of California then added their stamp of approval to the reasoning of the Court of Appeals and against the reasoning of Judge Allen. This jury was thereby ultimately and totally vindicated from all charges and accusations laid upon them by the trial judge. Unfortunately, it took two and a half long years after their verdict. In the end, they were clearly found to be "fair and impartial" as required by law and in accordance with their oath in their search for the truth.

Epilogue

The truth prevailed.

Unlike most product liability litigation which end in a confidential sealed settlement, rather than a judgment that is public, the "Pill" was now known to the entire world to cause thrombosis in some women.

Michelle and Dennis had accomplished their purpose.

The world now knew the real risks of taking the "Pill" so that women would now be able to exercise their right to choose for themselves whether to take such risks.

Had Michelle and Dennis been willing to compromise their claim along the way of litigation out of fear of losing, Johnson & Johnson, like the vast majority of manufacturers, would have insisted upon a settlement conditioned on absolute secrecy, and a request to the Court that the entire litigation evidence be sealed. There would have been be no access to any of the evidence we uncovered by either the press, other trial lawyers representing injured women from the "Pill," or the public at large.

The foregoing was dramatically illustrated three days following the *Ahearn* verdict in an extensive expose in a major East Coast newspaper, "The Record," at that time servicing most of New Jersey and New York State.

Using the *Ahearn* verdict as front page coverage with a large picture of Michelle alongside a packet of the "Pills," the headline read: "Settlements kept secret in Pill suits."

The article began:

> "A San Jose jury has awarded $1,248,000 to a California woman totally blinded by blood clots caused by the birth control pills. . . . It was the largest award on public record against a manufacturer of the pill. . . . The case was only the 23rd to go to trial among thousands of suits brought against the seven pill manufacturers across the country. . . . It highlights the success of pill manufacturers in keeping secret the thousands of cash settlements paid because women suffered blood clots, paralysis and even death, after using the pills."

The article continued with a two-page explanation of Big Pharma's tactics of secretly settling many "Pill" cases under court orders sealing all the facts and evidence involved. Such tactics deprived the general public, "Pill" victims, and their lawyers from becoming aware of, or having any access to, the powerful evidence uncovered in the settled cases. The seven pharmaceutical manufacturers of the "Pill" had utilized this tactic of secrecy for over ten years preceding the *Ahearn* verdict. Jerry Michaud, who hosted the critical Wichita brainstorming meeting and Paul Rheingold, an initial colleague in the *Ahearn* case, were a major source of the article's information on sealed settlements.

⊘

The jury verdict, itself, publicized in 1974 had already exposed the coverup and moved the pharmaceutical industry to properly warn of the thrombosis risk of the "Pill." Even the Court of Appeal's opinion noted in a footnote, that as early as late December 1974, (only weeks after the *Ahearn* verdict) a new revised and extensive warning label was issued for physicians which read, in part, as follows:

"Warnings

The use of oral contraceptives is associated with increased risk of several serious conditions including thromboembolism. . . . Practitioners prescribing oral contraceptives should be familiar with the following information relating to these risks.

1. Thromboembolic Disorders and Other Vascular Problems.

2. An increased risk of thromboembolic and thrombotic disease associated with the use of oral contraceptives is well established. . . .

3. Ocular Lesions. There have been reports of neuro-ocular lesions such as optic neuritis or

retinal thrombosis associated with the use of oral contraceptives. . . ."

Since that time, the warning of a cause and effect relationship between the "Pill" and thrombosis has continuously been strengthened. Today, there is no longer any ambiguity in the warnings regarding the "Pill" and thrombosis, nor any question of causation by anyone, including the medical world.

❧

From the evidence uncovered in the *Ahearn* case, the world now knows the pharmaceutical industry failed to do the proper pre-marketing testing that would have unveiled the risk of thrombosis. The world now knows Ortho further failed to properly communicate to physicians and the public the adverse reaction reports they were receiving daily. It now knows our regulatory agency, the FDA and its Advisory Committee, failed to stand up to the pressure of the industry and order adequate warnings of the existing "cause and effect" relationship between the "Pill" and thrombosis in a timely fashion. Only through this litigation was the world educated on the *truth* of the risk of thrombosis and the "Pill"—unfortunately years after it unnecessarily took too many young women's lives and caused too much human suffering.

❧

However, the persuasive power of product liability litigation exposure and the consequential effect of a powerful jury verdict upon industry accomplished even more. The pharmaceutical manufacturers finally studied what they should have done years before the "Pill" was ever marketed for use by the general public (1960). They initiated the necessary research to explore the efficacy of substantial reductions in the dosage of the ethinyl estradiol (estrogen component) in the "Pill," from its original content that Michelle was first prescribed, to a substantially lower dosage in today's "Pill." Despite the reduction, the "Pill" still maintains its same efficacy as an oral contraceptive to prevent pregnancies.

How many lives would have been saved, and how much human misery would have been avoided had this research been undertaken and completed *before* marketing to the public at large? Subsequent to the *Ahearn* litigation, many prescribing physicians have stated to me in one form or another, "You will never know the number of women's lives the *Ahearn* case has saved."

∞

Unfortunately, the *greed* of the pharmaceutical industry raised its ugly head in another way involving the "Pill." The *Ahearn* case made known to the world the clotting propensity of the "Pill" in *some women*. But, a woman's prescribing physician still had no known way of determining if a specific patient was among those susceptible to thrombosis when prescribed the "Pill," other than in situations of certain blood type variations, infection or trauma. That should *not* have been the case.

It was a completely unnecessary risk!

In the late 1970's, Harold discovered a medical article in the French literature describing an identifiable genetic factor that explained why only *some* women were susceptible to clotting, other than known blood type variations. The author, a French physician, had been doing extensive genetic research on arteriosclerotic disease in younger people. He seemed to have stumbled upon a specific gene variation that existed in 20% of the human race that rendered that person an increased risk for thrombosis when exposed to any blood clotting trigger, particularly the "Pill."

Harold and I were still litigating oral contraceptive cases at that time, so we had a definite interest in the work of this French Physician. Harold suggested we meet with Dr. Jean Louis Beaumont and learn more, so Harold made the first trip to Paris to meet with him. Harold returned very excited.

"Sal, you have to meet this man and see his work. He's found the answer to why only some women get thrombosis when on the 'Pill.'"

I was inspired by Harold's description of this scientist.

"Harold, would he be willing to see me as just an ordinary American lawyer, you're a physician?"

"He'll welcome you." Harold replied.

I flew to Paris. I arrived at a hospital, twenty miles outside of Paris where Dr. Beaumont maintained his office and research laboratory. I was escorted into his office to meet this extraordinary person who at the time was also a member of the French Parliament—a true Renaissance man.

As we shook hands, he explained that his English was sufficient for normal conversation, but when it came to medical terms, he preferred to use French. Since most medical terms in English are rooted in either Latin, German or French, I didn't feel this would be a problem because of my familiarity with medical terminology.

He devoted the entire day to educating me on his research and his findings.

I was astounded when he showed me a simple medical kit he had invented that would enable any physician to determine if a specific patient had this gene anomaly before prescribing the oral contraceptive. The physician and the patient would then know, before taking the "Pill," if she was more susceptible to blood clotting when exposed to the "Pill."

I asked if he had communicated this invaluable information to any American pharmaceutical manufacturers of the "Pill."

"Yes, definitely!" he said, and proceeded to pull from his files, copies of the actual letters he had sent Ortho, Searle, and others describing his work and his medical kit that would be a perfect solution to the problem.

After reading the letters, I asked him what was their reply since a substantial amount of time had elapsed since the letters had been sent?

He responded rather sadly, "There hasn't been any reply from any of them. They clearly are not interested."

I was aghast!

I thanked Dr. Beaumont for graciously devoting his entire day educating me on his work and asked if he would be willing to testify for me as an expert in my remaining "Pill" cases against these very manufacturers who failed to respond to the availability of his life saving kit. He agreed, so long as the timing of such trials were possible within his heavy schedule.

I pulled out my check book and asked how much I owed him for the many hours he gave me of his time. I was used to usually being charged for a physician's time when meeting with me.

Dr. Beaumont surprisingly said to me, "You can put your checkbook away. You do not owe me anything. As I do my work with the hope of saving lives through medicine, you do your work to save lives through the law. I do not want to be paid by you."

I was astounded that this masterful French physician, scientist, and member of the French Parliament would be so gracious to an American trial lawyer.

As I flew home, I thought to myself, *why wouldn't the pharmaceutical manufacturers of the "Pill" want to make Dr. Beaumont's life-saving kit available to the medical world?*

The only answer that became quite obvious was that if 20% of young women of childbearing age could not be prescribed the "Pill" because of this kit identifying their gene anomaly, the pharmaceutical manufacturers of the "Pill" would automatically lose 20% of their sales. Big Pharma greed continued to control their decisions—and the *greed* continues. Since our subsequent cases ultimately resolved through settlements without the necessity of trials, it was unfortunately never necessary to call upon Dr. Beaumont for his testimony.

✑

After suffering through this long ordeal, Michelle and Dennis attempted to return to their normal daily lives, Dennis as a successful architectural engineer, and Michelle as the caring wife and mother of three children. But it could never be normal for either of them again. Though satisfied they were ultimately successful in getting justice, no amount of money in the world could replace living the rest of their lives dealing with Michelle's permanent lasting blindness. However, their courage to deal with the future did not wane one bit.

Michelle's adjustments in carrying on with the many other duties of life did not come easy, nor would it for any human being. To handle all the chores of being a mother of three young children, cooking, cleaning, rendering the necessary discipline, all the while living with the loneliness of a dark world takes incredible courage and determination. Yet, she did it courageously and well. Her children are now grown, and family responsibilities have lessened. She now enjoys grandchildren who, of course, she has never seen. Dennis and Michelle continue to adjust to aging and retirement. Her memory of this case, however, lives on as though it was yesterday.

✑

One would expect that having reversed Judge Allen on such a major case, he would not be very friendly toward me thereafter. Nothing could have been further from the truth. He was respectful toward me in future cases when appearing before him and very fair in his rulings on such cases. He ruled in my favor on another oral contraceptive case against Searle, another "Pill" manufacturer, ordering them to give me access to their entire document file on their product.

Years later, Judge Allen and I worked together on a special committee created to study and recommend whether Municipal Courts should be merged into the Superior Courts of Santa Clara County so as to create a single court system throughout the County, and eventually the entire state of California. We worked well together, both reaching the same conclusion with the majority of the committee that the courts should be merged into one system. That he not only failed to hold a grudge against me, but rather respected my competence as a lawyer became quite apparent years later when he referred a close family member to retain me to represent them in a personal injury auto accident case.

Judge Allen has since deceased as have most of the major characters in this real-life story.

∾

A short time after the *Ahearn* case came to an end, Harold Williams moved to California and joined our firm. We worked together on many cases on complex medical issues during that time. He subsequently retired to the beautiful northern California coast. He passed away in 2013 at the age of 92.

∾

A year after the *Ahearn* case was over, I received an unusual phone call that led to the disclosure of a secret strategy employed by Johnson & Johnson in the case. He was an insurance claims person with whom I had professional dealings over several years.

"Sal, my employer has just laid me off so I'm free to talk with you now about things that occurred in the *Ahearn* case, that I'm sure you're completely unaware of. How about having lunch sometime this week?"

I was immediately intrigued. He piqued my curiosity, so I said, "How about tomorrow?"

We met the next day at a local restaurant and after exchanging the usual pleasantries, he opened the subject matter with a question.

"Sal, where did you get the money to finance the *Ahearn* case? Ortho tried everything they could to bankrupt you."

I assumed he was referring to the lack of people to assist me in the case, so I replied somewhat jokingly, but not entirely, "Ortho overlooked my capacity to skip sleep at night and work twenty-four hours a day."

He told the story of how the insurance company for whom he had been employed was working with Ortho on their defense in the *Ahearn* case. He described several strategy meetings he attended in which my personal financial strength to proceed through the litigation to its end was a significant subject of discussion. He described how they had ordered a thorough investigation into my financial status and knew that I, alone, was financing the case. They discussed ways of deliberately increasing the financial strain on me through the litigation discovery procedures with the goal of "bankrupting" me before the case could be brought to trial.

⁂

Following the conclusion of the *Ahearn* case, my original partner, Dick Caputo, and I were able to expand our firm to as many as 25 lawyers and over 100 employees, with several lawyers working with us in the field of tort liability, and particularly in the trial of product liability cases. In addition to personal injury cases, I continued to handle oral contraceptive cases until the early 1980's when my focus changed to other product cases, many of which continued to involve a woman's right to know.

Dick retired from the firm in the early 1990's. The firm disbanded in the early 2000's and I downsized my personal injury/product liability trial practice. More recently my focus has turned to mediation, arbitration, consulting for trial lawyers, and, of course, writing.

Finally, I would be remiss if I failed to admit that certain powerful words that arose from this story shall never be forgotten. They are the words spoken as a sincere belief by a renowned, courageous pharmacologist at the risk of his entire career—spoken to a young trial lawyer in whom he was willing to place great trust.

"The oral contraceptive is the biggest fraud ever perpetuated upon American Womanhood."

This physician's overriding belief in a woman's right to know could not have been stated any clearer. I was proud to have proven in the courts of law the truth of those powerful words.

Afterword

Lessons to be taken away from this factual historical event are many.

The most critical in my mind is the value to our legal system of trial by jury. Trial by jury under our system of justice allows lay jurors from different walks of life to possess the capacity and authority under our laws to overcome even inaccurate evidentiary findings of a trial judge. They have the power and authority under the law to reach the truth against a Goliath American Corporation. They possess the power to hold such a Goliath publicly accountable for its misdeeds motivated by greed and pay for the consequences of its *conduct placing profits over human life*.

Many people view product liability litigation as an expression of the "greed" of plaintiff trial lawyers. Nothing could be further from the truth, as clearly demonstrated in the *Ahearn* saga. Counting all the hours, days, weeks, months, and years of demanding work (total of eight years), against all odds, the extensive time away from my family, the substantial financial risk demanded by this case, at the end of the day, my wife calculated that my hourly compensation in the *Ahearn* case was well below the minimum wage.

As a profession, many plaintiff trial lawyers, particularly those in product liability work, are motivated more by the desire and challenge to create a safer world than by any enticement of money alone. That fact, unfortunately, never makes the headlines of the local newspaper or newscast, and either is unknown, or readily escapes the attention of the general public.

Our jury system has become unique in this aspect and one that must be protected, for as we have seen in this story, the influence of Big Pharma can even reach into the FDA preventing the truth from reaching physicians, as well as the public. We must preserve the jury system at all cost against the continuous daily attacks from the insurance industry, pharmaceutical industry, and the entire industrial world.

As seen in the "Pill" litigation, product safety devices and warnings that save lives and prevent injuries, ranging from automobiles to prescription drugs, more often than not, originated with a product liability lawsuit being filed by an injured plaintiff, and the verdicts that followed from conscientious juries performing their duty.

Several years ago, I researched the origin of many modern safety devices and changes in automobile design for a lecture to trial lawyers on the value to society of product liability litigation. Not surprisingly, I found an Appellate Court decision upholding a jury verdict preceded each major highway safety standard that brought about such safety changes.

It is the *rule of law* exercised through the advocacy nature of product litigation that bears the greatest credit for product safety in America today. Many examples abound in our product history such as: infection causing IUDs, exploding gas tank designs, the introduction of safe seatbelts, air bags, anti-skid brakes, crush absorbing designs in automobiles, anti-inflammatory materials used in airplanes and clothing, specific warnings on most prescriptive drugs, roll-over prevention design on automobiles, tractors, and even golf carts. Today, there exists an unending list of common products safely used in everyday life that are the result of such litigation. Behind these safety devices and warnings are years of intense litigation, handled by trial lawyers all over America, on behalf of their injured or deceased clients, similar to this case.

Even as I am in the process of finishing this story on the *Ahearn* case, Johnson & Johnson's continued greed has resulted in a $37 million-dollar verdict for general damages, and an $80 million-dollar punitive damage verdict against them and their talc supplier. This courageous New Jersey jury, seeking the truth, found that this pharmaceutical giant acted with reckless indifference in selling *asbestos-containing talcum powder* that contributed to a man's development of mesothelioma, a fatal lung disease. In another case, a Pennsylvania appeals court threw out an order that had kept a Johnson & Johnson subsidiary from facing punitive damages in thousands of cases pending in Philadelphia County. The victim plaintiffs were young boys who developed breasts after taking the antipsychotic medication Risperdal. As recent as January 31, 2019, a Philadelphia jury returned a verdict against a Johnson & Johnson subsidiary, Ethicon, Inc., in the amount of $41 million. The jury found that defects in a pelvic mesh implant manufactured by the company had caused a woman permanent injuries when the product sawed into her vagina.

✑

A museum of some of these history-making cases was established by Ralph Nader a few years ago with major contributions by many of the great trial lawyers of the time. The purpose was to provide a history illustrating tort cases that have made this world a safer place in which to live. The American Museum of Tort Law is located in Winsted, Connecticut.

✑

The only available weapon to the injured and trial lawyer in their continued quest to increase safety in our daily lives—is the Rule of Law. Fortunately, for all Americans in the United States of America today, the search for the truth through our courts of law continues.

Newspaper Articles

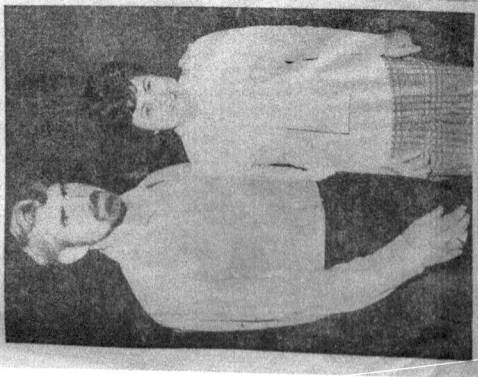

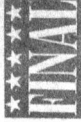

San Jose Mercury, December 17, 1974

BIRTH CONTROL PILL SUIT

Blinded S.J. Wife Wins $1.1 Million

By GEORGE NEWMAN
Staff Writer

A nine-woman, three-man jury Monday awarded $1,142,586 in damages to a 35-year-old San Jose housewife who went blind after taking Ortho-Novum birth-control pills.

Mrs. Michelle Ahearn of 3370 Cardin Ave., mother of three children, removed her dark glasses, burst into tears and sobbed uncontrollably for several minutes when she heard the verdict.

Moments later, the jury awarded $105,668 in damages to her husband, Dennis, a structural engineer.

He, too, began to cry softly and put his arm around his wife.

As the jurors filed out of the courtroom, nearly every one embraced Mrs. Ahearn. She said "thank you so much" to each and wished them a "wonderful Christmas."

Her husband said the verdict "will allow Michelle her independence."

"I won't have to depend on my children (now ages 8 to 14) in my old age," Mrs. Ahearn said.

The verdicts concluded a trial that began Oct. 31 in the Santa Clara County Superior Courtroom of Judge Bruce F. Allen.

They were directed at all three defendants: the Ortho Pharmaceutical Co., which manufactures the pill, and its parent company, Johnson & Johnson, and Lucky Stores, owner of the Gemco pharmacy and its parent company, Johnson Johnson, where Mrs. Ahearn bought the pills.

The physician who prescribed Ortho-Novum was not named as a defendant.

According to testimony,

Mrs. Ahearn began taking Ortho-Novum in 1967 on her doctor's prescription. She said she suffered periodic headaches while taking the pills into 1969.

On Feb. 15, 1969, she testified, she started to experience the onset of severe headaches and blindness.

Three days later, physicians testified, Mrs. Ahearn

(Back of Section, Col. 2)

Blind Wife Wins Birth Pills Suit

(Continued from Page 1)

was totally blind and the blindness was permanent.

Doctors said her blindness was caused by clots which blocked the supply of blood to her optic nerves. This caused them to atrophy and die from lack of blood and oxygen, they said.

Defense attorney M.J. Pothoven of Sacramento contended unsuccessfully that Mrs. Ahearn was suffering from a streptococcus infection at the time which caused the clotting.

Mrs. Ahearn's attorneys, Sal Liccardo of San Jose and Dr. J. Harold Williams, a medical doctor and attorney from Wichita, Kan., charged that the blindness was caused either by the pill by itself or by a combination of the pill and the infection.

The total verdict for the Ahearns came to $1,248,254.

Eighteen medical specialists from across the nation testified at the trial.

Williams said he travels almost exclusively trying birth-control pill cases.

He said he recently assisted in another Ortho-Novum trial for a woman who suffered blindness in one eye.

He said she was awarded $280,000 in damages and the verdict recently was upheld by the Oregon State Supreme Court.

San Jose Mercury, December 17, 1974—Continued

S.J. Woman Made Blind By Pill Wins $1.1 Million

A tearful San Jose housewife who says she was blinded by birth control pills wished her lawsuit jurors "a wonderful Christmas" after they granted her $1.1 million in damages.

Mrs. Michelle Ahearn, wife of structural engineer Dennis Ahearn, 3370 Cardin Ave., burst into tears moments after the verdict was read Monday in Santa Clara County Superior Court.

The blinded 35-year-old housewife and mother of three said the verdict means that "I won't have to depend on my children in my old age."

Hit by the decision was the Johnson & Johnson Co., which owns Ortho Pharmaceutical Co., manufacturer of Ortho-Novum, the birth control pill which Mrs. Ahearn says blinded her.

Lucky Stores, which owns Gemco pharmacy, where Mrs. Ahearn bought the pills, was named in the suit along with the pharmacy.

According to testimony, Mrs. Ahearn began taking the pill in 1967 and suffered periodic headaches.

On Feb. 15, 1969, she began feeling more headaches while at the same time experiencing blindness. Three days later she was totally blind.

Doctors said her blindness was caused by clots which blocked the blood supply to her optic nerves, causing them to atrophy and die.

Defense attorneys contended that the blindness was caused by a streptococcus infection. Mrs. Ahearn's attorneys said that blindness

(Back of Section, Col. 1)

SAN JOSE NEWS

Vol. 183, No. 126, 92nd Year ★★★★★ SAN JOSE, CA., TUES., DEC. 17, 1974 70 Pages 15 Cents

San Jose News, December 17, 1974

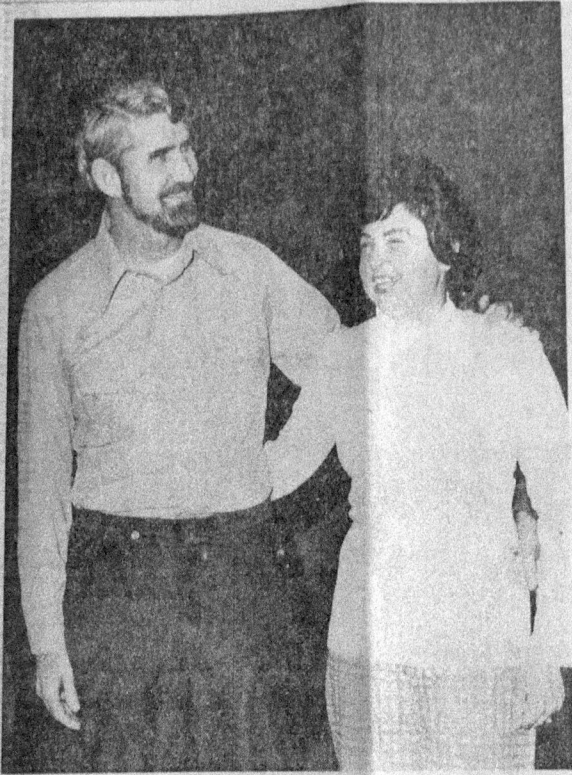

20 Tues., Dec. 17, 1974 ★★★★★ San Jose News

DENNIS, MICHELLE AHEARN . . . Happy After Superior Court Jury Announced Verdicts

—Staff Photo

S.J. Woman Made Blind By Pill Wins $1.1 Million

(Continued from Page 1) was caused either by the pill or by a combination of the pill and the infection.

Total verdict came to $1,-248,254, with $105,668 awarded in damages to Mrs. Ahearn's husband, who said

the verdict "will allow Michelle her independence."

Testifying in the case for Mrs. Ahearn was Dr. J. Harold Williams, also an attorney, who said he travels almost exclusively trying birth control pill cases.

Mrs. Ahearn's attorneys were Sal Liccardo of San Jose and Dr. Williams. The defense attorney was M.J. Pothoven.

The trial took place in the courtroom of Superior Judge Bruce F. Allen.

San Jose News, December 17, 1974—Continued

San Francisco Examiner

10th Year No. 162   ★ 2R   TUESDAY, DECEMBER 17, 1974   DAILY 20¢

Blinded, she gets million in pill suit

By Don West
Examiner News Staff

SAN JOSE — A jury has awarded a San Jose mother more than $1 million in damages on the ground that she became blind after taking a widely-used birth-control pill.

The verdict awarded $1,-142,586 to Mrs. Michelle Ahearn, 35. Her husband Dennis, a structural engineer, was awarded $105,668.

The drug at issue is Ortho-Novum, one of the most widely prescribed of the oral contraceptives. The defendants were the manufacturers — Ortho Pharmaceutical Co. and its parent company, Johnson & Johnson of New Brunswick, N. J. — and Lucky Stores, owners of the Gemco Pharmacy where she bought the pills.

The suit did not name the physician who prescribed the drug.

Mrs. Ahearn, mother of three, said she began taking the pills in 1967 and continued until 1969. She testified she suffered headaches and severe nausea, and on Feb. 16, 1969, began losing her sight.

During the trial of her suit before Superior Court Judge Bruce Allen, medical witnesses for Mrs. Ahearn testified her blindness was caused by clots that blocked blood circulation to the optic nerves.

This deprived them of needed oxygen and caused them to atrophy and die, according to the testimony. The mother was described as permanently blind.

San Francisco Examiner, December 17, 1974

San Francisco Chronicle

The Largest Daily Circulation in Northern California

★★★★ WEDNESDAY, DECEMBER 18, 1974 GArti

$1.1 Million Award in Pill Suit

A San Jose housewife who became permanently blind in both eyes while taking birth control pills has been awarded more than $1 million in damages.

The manufacturer of the pills maintained after the trial that its products were not to blame and said it will appeal the decision.

The unanimous nine-woman, three-man Santa Clara county Superior Court jury also awarded $105,668 to the woman's husband for loss of her services.

Both Michelle Ahearn, 35, and her husband, Dennis, a structural engineer, of 3370 Cardin avenue, wept upon learning the verdict Monday.

According to testimony, Mrs. Ahearn, mother of three, who had been taking Ortho-Novum for two years on a doctor's prescription, began suffering severe headaches in 1969 that led immediately to permanent bilateral blindness.

Several doctors testified the blindness was caused by clots that stopped the flow of blood to the woman's optic nerves, which atrophied

The defense contended Mrs. Ahearn suffered a streptococcus infection that caused the clotting, but the jury held that the pill was a significant contributing fac-

Back Page Col. 5

San Francisco Chronicle, December 18, 1974

BIRTH PILL SUIT

From Page 1

tor in the blindness.

The $1,142,586 awarded to Mrs. Ahearn is one of the largest amounts ever given in a suit involving negligence and breach of warranty.

The award went against the Ortho Pharmaceutical Co., the manufacturer, its parent company, Johnson and Johnson, and Lucky Stores, the retail distributor.

An official at Johnson and Johnson, reached at the corporate headquarters in New Brunswick, N. J., said after the trial, "Of course, we will appeal. We feel the medical testimony presented at the trial clearly established that the blindness was caused by an infection. Our product, we feel, was not implicated."

Mrs. Ahearn's attorney, Sal Liccardo of San Jose, refused to divulge his fees in the case.

Eighteen medical witnesses, several from out of state, testified during the six-week trial.

Several local researchers were asked yesterday, in light of the trial, what women now taking Ortho-Novum or other oral contraceptives should conclude.

"This brand is no more or less dangerous than others," said Dr. Sumner Kalman, a professor of pharmacology at Stanford University. "Women taking the pill shouldn't conclude from this that they will be blinded."

However, he said, studies in the ten years since the pill came into widespread use have convincingly demonstrated an increase in blood clots among women taking it.

The chances of "serious" blood clots, requiring medical attention, increase among young women using

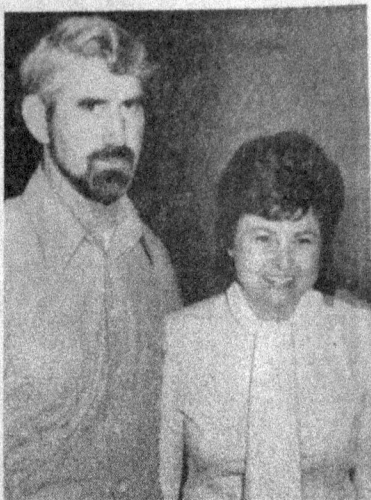

AP Wirephoto

DENNIS AND MICHELLE AHEARN
She lost her sight while taking the pills

the pill to three in 100,000 per year, compared to the norm of one per 100,000.

"This is still a pretty small risk," said Kalman.

There are some signs to look for to warn of possible blood clot problems, he added.

Among them are pain in the lower extremities, cough or pain in the chest, and severe headaches. If these occur, the women taking the pill should check with their doctors, Kalman said.

Dr. Neil Raskin, associate professor of neurology at the University of California Medical Center here, said headaches in particular should be an indication not to use the pill.

"There is clear evidence that strokes occur more frequently among young women using the pill than those not using it," he said. "One of the theories is that the

strokes are caused by mechanisms similar to what causes migraine headaches — constriction of blood vessels in the brain. The pill can aggravate this condition, and a stroke can cause a lot of problems, including blindness."

Kalman said he personally does not recommend long-term use of the pill "simply because it is a powerful drug whose exact mode of action we don't understand. It is suppressing some very important mechanisms of ovulation.

"In particular, any woman with a history of migraine or heavy headaches should not use oral contraceptives.

"However, the risk is still small, and some women will still want to use the pill. The law requires the risks and side effects to be listed in a package insert with the pills. They are all there."

$1-Million in Birth Pill Suit

SAN JOSE, Calif., Dec. 17 (UPI)—Mrs. Michelle Ahearn, 35 years old, and her husband, Dennis, have been awarded more than $1-million damages in a suit over birth control pills that she said made her permanently blind. A Santa Clara County Superior Court jury awarded the woman $1,248,254 and her husband $105,668. The defendants were the Ortho Pharmaceutical Company, manufacturer of Ortho-Novum, the Johnson & Johnson Drug Company, and Lucky Stores, owner of the pharmacy where the drug was purchased on a prescription.

The New York Times
Published: December 18, 1974

New York Times, December 18, 1974

Los Angeles Times

WEDNESDAY MORNING, DECEMBER 18, 1974

THE STATE

Woman Blinded by Pills Wins $1.14 Million

Ortho-Novum birth control pills contributed to the blindness of a 35-year-old San Jose woman, a jury declared in awarding her $1.14 million.

Michelle Ahearn said she began taking the pills in 1967 and went blind in 1969. Doctors said clots blocked the blood suppy to her optic nerves, and the nerves therefore died, causing Mrs. Ahearn to lose her sight. Jurors in the court of Superior Judge Bruce F. Allen also awarded Mrs. Ahearn's husband, Dennis, $105,668. Both verdicts were directed against the Ortho Pharmaceutical Co., its parent company, Johnson & Johnson, and Lucky Stores, owner of the Gemco pharmacy where Mrs. Ahearn bought the pills.

Los Angeles Times, December 18, 1974

10 THE WALL STREET JOURNAL,
Wednesday, Dec. 18, 1974

Johnson & Johnson Loses Damage Suit On Birth Control Pills

SAN JOSE, Calif.—(AP)—A 35-year-old woman, blinded after taking birth control pills, was awarded $1.1 million in damages by a superior court jury.

Michelle Ahearn of San Jose was awarded damages after a seven-week trial. Her husband, Dennis, was awarded $105,668 in damages.

Both verdicts were directed against Ortho Pharmaceutical Corp., maker of Ortho-Novum birth control pills, and its parent company, Johnson & Johnson. Lucky Stores, owner of the Gemco pharmacy where Mrs. Ahearn bought the pills, also was held liable.

(An Ortho spokesman said the company would appeal the decision. "The medical evidence presented at the trial, in the company's judgment, proved that Mrs. Ahearn's blindness was caused by a streptococcal infection and had no direct or indirect relationship to her use of oral contraceptives," the spokesman said.)

(In Dublin, Calif., an official of Lucky Stores said the company wasn't a party in the lawsuit and isn't liable for any of the damage award, and thus can't comment on the decision.)

Mrs. Ahearn started taking the pills under a doctor's prescription in 1967. She testified that in February 1969 she had severe headaches and the onset of blindness. Doctors said she became totally blind within three days and that the condition was permanent.

The blindness was caused by clots that blocked blood supply to the optic nerves, which died because of lack of blood and oxygen, doctors said.

(This is the second recent judgment against Ortho. In November, the Oregon Supreme Court confirmed the award of $280,978 in damages to a Portland woman who claimed she lost the sight of one eye after taking oral contraceptives made by Ortho and Syntex Corp. of Palo Alto, Calif.

(Confirming a lower court decision, the Oregon court ruled that Ortho and Syntex were liable for damages because they didn't provide "timely, adequate warnings to the medical profession" about possible dangerous side effects.

(Labels accompanying all birth control pills routinely warn of the increased possibility of health-endangering blood clots in women taking oral contraceptives.)

Wall Street Journal, December 18, 1974

THE WEST AUSTRALIAN THURSDAY DECEMBER 19 1974 **21**

PILL BLINDS: $860,000 AWARD

LOS ANGELES, Wed: A 35-year-old woman blinded after taking birth control pills, has been awarded $A860,000 in damages by a Superior Court jury.

Mrs Michelle Ahearn, of San Jose, California, was awarded damages yesterday after a seven-week trial before Judge Bruce Allen. Mrs Ahearn's husband, Dennis, was awarded $80,000 damages.

Both verdicts were di-rected against Ortho Pharmaceutical Co., man-ufacturer of Ortho-Novum birth control pills, and its parent company, Johnson and Johnson.

Lucky Stores, owner of the Gemco pharmacy where Mrs Ahearn bought the pills, also was held liable.

The mother of three children took off her dark glasses and sobbed uncontrollably for sever-al minutes when the ver-dict was read. Her hus-band put his arm around her and cried softly. Most of the jurors em-braced Mrs Ahearn as they filed out of the court.

Mrs Ahearn started tak-ing the pills under a doc-tor's prescription in 1967. She testified that in Feb-ruary 1969 she exper-ienced severe headaches and the onset of blind-ness. Doctors said she be-came totally blind within three days, and the con-dition was permanent.

The blindness was caused by clots that blocked blood supply to the optic nerves, which died because of lack of blood and oxygen, the doctors said.

The drug firm main-tained that the clots were caused by a strepto-coccus infection and not by the pill. Dr Harold Williams, a physician and attorney who repre-sented the Ahearns, argued that the blindness resulted from use of the pill or a combination of the pill and the infection. —AAP.

Ortho Pharmaceutical Corporation

RARITAN · NEW JERSEY 08869

Dear Doctor:

Ortho Pharmaceutical Corporation has just completed a seven week trial in San Jose, California in which a woman alleged that ORTHO-NOVUM* Tablets caused her to become blind. The plaintiff presented medical testimony supporting this allegation. The jury returned a verdict in favor of the plaintiff and awarded her $1.3 million in damages. We plan to appeal this decision.

Because of the nature of the case, it has received wide publicity in the media and we want you to know the facts in the case which we feel were not accepted by the jury in reaching its verdict.

The patient in question was hospitalized with a bilateral orbital cellulitis, a septicemia with beta hemolytic streptococci and meningitis. During the course of this illness, she was found to be blind in both eyes. The above infectious disease is a well recognized condition which historically has resulted in blindness. It is our opinion and that of the treating physicians as well as other highly qualified medical experts that the oral contraceptive had nothing to do with her blindness, and for this reason, as stated previously, we are going to appeal this case to a higher court.

Because of the extensive publicity, your office may be receiving telephone calls regarding the case. The above information is presented so that you have a more complete understanding of the circumstances in this case.

                                        Ortho Pharmaceutical Corporation

*Trademark

Ortho's Letter to Physicians After Verdict

The Record

Friend of the People It Serves

Vol. 80 — No. 166   92 PAGES — Four Sections   WEDNESDAY, DECEMBER 18, 1974

Birth-control pills (dispenser is shown at left) are leading to lawsuits. Woman blinded by pill reaction smiles after jury award; most suits are settled privately and secretly.

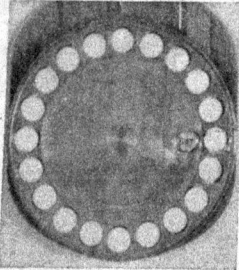

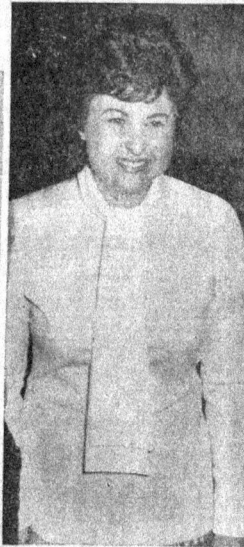

Settlements kept secret in pill suits

By ANN CRAWFORD
Staff Writer

A San Jose grand jury has awarded $1,340,000 to a young California woman totally blinded by blood clots caused by birth control pills. It was the largest award on public record against a manufacturer of the pills.

The award was made Monday to Mrs. Michelle Ahearne, who took pills manufactured by Ortho Pharmaceutical Division of Johnson & Johnson, New Brunswick.

The case was only the 33rd to go to trial among thousands of suits brought against the seven pill manufacturers across the country. It highlights the success of pill manufacturers in keeping secret the thousands of cash settlements paid because women suffered blood clots, paralysis, and even death after using the pills.

Two courtroom devices are being used. Drug company lawyers are insisting that plaintiffs and their lawyers sign secrecy agreements as a precondition to cash settlements. More recently, the companies have prevailed on plaintiffs and judges to hide from public scrutiny all the documents in such cases, including the settlements.

Sealing criticized

The second device, called "sealing the file," has drawn criticism from constitutional and public-interest lawyers.

On Dec. 2, U.S. District Court Chief Judge Lawrence A. Whipple in Newark sealed the file in a suit against G.D. Searle Co. of Skokie, Ill., developer of the pill in 1960 and defendant in an estimated 40 percent of pill suits. The judge's law clerks explain the sealing was to expedite a settlement.

As a result, the only things the public can learn about the case are that Willie Gray, administrator of his wife's estate, brought suit in 1970 against Searle, Planned Parenthood, and Dr. Nadia Convalus; the

See PILL, Page A-2

The Record, December 18, 1974

Pill lawsuits covered up

From Page A-1

names of their lawyers; the names of jurors chosen in chambers on Dec. 2; the fact that a settlement was reached before testimony began and that the settlement and the entire file were sealed by the judge.

Major facts concealed

The public probably will never know if it was claimed that Mrs. Gray died as a result of using Searle's birth control pill, what settlement was agreed to, or whether Planned Parenthood and the doctor were involved in the settlement.

Also concealed were the nature of Mrs. Gray's symptoms, the way her husband's lawyers planned to prove the pill was the cause, the names of expert witnesses on both sides, and the company's own records on adverse effects of its oral contraceptives.

Gerald L. Michaud, a Wichita lawyer specializing in medical cases, explained why such secrecy is sought by pharmaceutical houses. Michaud's firm has filed 96 suits against the seven present or former manufacturers of the pill.

The purpose of the secrecy is to keep the public from knowing the problems associated with the pill," Michaud said. "When we see 100 cases filed, and know there is going to be no publicity, we know there are 1,000 people who have had things happen, but are not aware of the possible connection with the pill.

"When people read about the suits," he continued, "they become more conscious of the possible connection and seek legal remedy.

'Proof is big problem'

"Proof of causation is the big problem, and the defendants don't want lawyers exchanging information on their cases and on the methods used by successful lawyers."

Especially ticklish, Michaud said, is data his firm has obtained under court order directly from pharmaceutical company files.

To get over the secrecy hurdle, lawyers representing women with claims of birth control pill injuries have or-

ganized informally. Michaud's firm has conducted seminars on pill problems. Another lawyers' information clearinghouse is the so-called Pill Group organized by New York attorney Paul Rheingold.

Rheingold said he frequently encountered the secrecy agreement and was finding a growing number of judges who would consent to sealing whole files.

High stakes in secrecy

"We recently settled a case that way in a New Jersey state court," Rheingold said. "When the problem [of secrecy] is posed, it means extra thousands of dollars to your client and you can't say 'no'."

The settlement offered in return for secrecy is too large to resist, he explained.

Rheingold said there are thousands of such suits across the country, many of them being settled successfully.

Michaud reported personal knowledge of 2,000 suits and speculated there was as many more he didn't know of. Half a dozen other lawyers interviewed confirmed the estimates and the secrecy arrangements. They would not allow use of their names because they have cases pending or because they are under court order not to discuss their cases.

Reports on adverse effects

Michaud said his explorations of company files have shown thousands of reports of adverse effects. "For every one reported," he said, "there are probably many times that number that go unreported by doctors or unrecognized."

Until Monday, only 22 pill cases had been publicly tried. They have involved all seven manufacturers. Company defendants have won 7 out of 10 trials because of the difficulty of proving the pill caused the injuries, Rheingold said.

Searle's legal counsel, Roger Theis, refused to say how many suits have been brought against Searle or to talk about settlement figures. The Pharmaceutical Manufacturers Association in Washington confirmed that this silence was industry practice.

Theis did confirm that many of his company's pill cases are sealed in both state and federal courts. Sometimes, he said, secrecy arrangements were sought by plaintiffs' lawyers

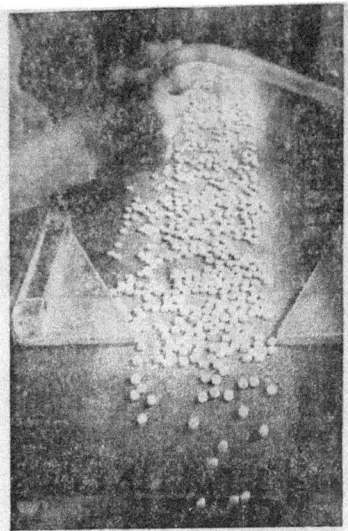

Some of the millions of birth control pills made yearly.

who didn't want colleagues to know they had accepted small settlements.

All plaintiffs' lawyers interviewed objected to the sealing procedure, some saying they had never heard of it and doubted its legality.

Calls it legal but undesirable

Cyril C. Means Jr., professor of constitutional law at New York Law School, said he doubted a constitutional attack could be made against the sealing but called it highly undesirable.

"The efficiency of the pills is a matter of great public interest," he said. "The moral right of the public to know looms large."

Anita Johnson, a lawyer at Ralph Nader's Health Research Group in Washington, called it outrageous. Publication of settlements serves to inform pill users and their families that they might be entitled to damages if they suffered ill effects, she said.

Law clerks for Judge Whipple said the sealing was agreed to to prevent a domino effect because of the large number of birth control suits pending. Publication of settlements might provoke other, perhaps unjustified settlements, they theorized.

The clerks said the sealing of the Gray suit did not constitute policy for federal courts in New Jersey despite the fact that Whipple is chief judge.

'Court doing its job'

"Policy in this and all courts is to promote settlements," one clerk said. "The court was doing its job in set-

tling this case. If there are adverse effects on society, that is for the legislative branch to cure."

Searle has settled three recent cases in Newark Federal Court and has at least two more pending. There are 90 federal district courts in the United States.

Other pill manufacturers were Parke-Davis Inc., Wyeth Laboratories Division of American Home Products Corp., Ortho Pharmaceutical Division of Johnson & Johnson, Upjohn Co., and Mead Johnson & Co. Upjohn and Mead Johnson no longer sell the pill.

The current strength of the pill is about one tenth that of the original 1960 pill. Specialists say the lower dosage has diminished the number of women who have adverse effects but not the seriousness of the injuries in those affected.

Though all seven manufacturers are publicly owned companies, subject to the financial reporting requirements of the Securities & Exchange Commission, they escape reporting all but the most general information about negligence suits.

A loophole in SEC regulations says the suits need not be reported if they are covered by insurance.

The Record, December 18, 1974—Continued

The Mercury

★★★★ SAN JOSE, CALIF., TUESDAY MORNING, DECEMBER 24, 1974   13

FIGURE IN $1-MILLION SUIT

Women Warned On The Pill

The public and the medical profession still haven't been told the full truth about birth-control pills.

So says Dr. J. Harold Williams, the doctor-lawyer from Wichita, Kans., who helped a San Jose housewife win $1.1 million in damages for blindness assertedly caused by the pill.

The pill is less dangerous now because the estrogen levels have been cut down, according to Dr. Williams.

"But blood clots still may occur," he said, "and the language of the pill warning is watered down."

In a telephone interview from his Wichita home, Williams said:

"I'm not against birth control pills or fertility pills if people are aware of the dangers they face while using them.

"But I think you should say, 'It's not nice to fool with mother nature.'"

In this era of "meddlesome medicine," Williams declared:

"We're fussing around with normal, healthy young women's physiologies and we don't know how many serious problems we may have in the future."

Williams joined Attorney Sal Liccardo of San Jose in successfully prosecuting the case of Mrs. Michelle Ahearn, 35, of 3370 Cardin Ave.

Mrs. Ahearn went blind after taking Ortho-Novum birth-control pills.

The birth-control warning required by the Federal Drug Administration (FDA) since 1970, "came too late for Mrs. Ahearn," said Dr. Williams.

The mother of three children testified the pills she had been taking on her doctor's prescription since 1967 gave her periodic headaches that became more severe, finally ending in blindness in 1969.

The Mercury, December 24, 1974

38   Friday, Jan. 3, 1975 ★★★ San Jose News

Moratorium On 'The Pill' Urged By Doctors' Union

A local physician's union has started a drive to stop doctors from prescribing birth control pills.

Dr. William Vederman, president of Local 7402 of the Union of American Physicians, said Thursday his group will launch a moratorium against prescribing the pills, and encourage other medical societies to follow suit. The union local says it represents approximately 15 per cent of the practicing physicians in Santa Clara County.

Vederman said his group is not against birth control, "but prescription of pills is legally untenable."

LAWSUIT

Vederman said the drive was motivated by the recent lawsuit brought by San Jose housewife Michelle Ahearn, 3370 Cardin Ave. Mrs. Ahearn was awarded more than $1.1 million in damages after she allegedly went blind as the result of taking Ortho-Novum birth control pills.

The jury ruled against the Ortho Pharmaceutical Company, its parent company, Johnson & Johnson, and Lucky Stores, owner of the Gemco pharmacy where Mrs. Ahearn bought the pills.

Mrs. Ahearn's physician was not named in the lawsuit, but according to Vederman "it's only because he has extremely good rapport with his patient."

Vederman claims doctors are becoming paranoid about the threat of malpractice suits, and that many are leary of prescribing "the Pill."

One local gynecologist, Dr. Bert Johnson, said he probably would not prescribe any more birth control pills "unless we get some legislative relief."

Johson said, "The Pill is actually the most effective and best method available for family planning. On a statistical basis, it is the safest of all contraceptive measures."

"But if side-effects from the Pill could cause me to be slapped with a million dollar lawsuit, I'm going to be very apprehensive about prescribing it."

Vederman laid the blame directly to lawyers and to money-motivated patients.

GET RICH

"This (malpractice) has become a plum for a small number of patients who see it as a way to get rich quick," he said.

"And the enormous contingency fees in some of the cases we've seen don't give anyone with power to make changes, the incentive to make changes."

"Legislators are led to believe that these huge sums are justified," he said. "We are hoping to put pressure on lawyers to change things."

Vederman said his group is beginning a drive for support countywide, but hopes to drum up enthusiasm across the state and perhaps the nation.

"We're attempting to accomplish a realignment of the malpractice situation," he said. "It's not to deprive patients of birth control, which they require. We're talking about the elective prescription of birth control pills."

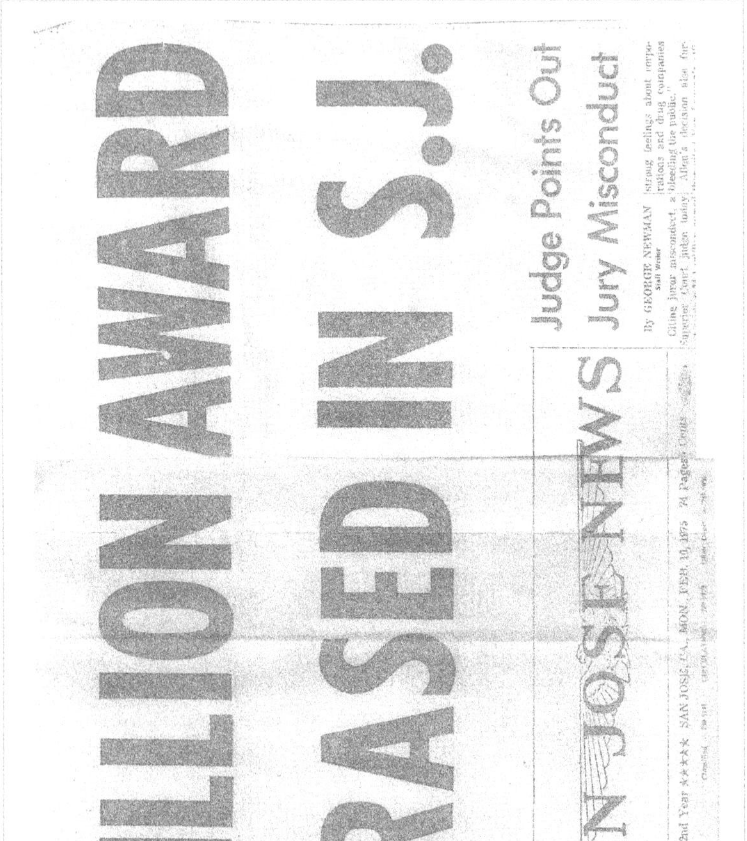

$1.1 MILLION AWARD ERASED IN S.J.

SPORTS FINAL

SAN JOSE NEWS

Vol. 184, No. 17, 92nd Year ★★★★★ SAN JOSE, CA., MON., FEB. 10, 1975 74 Pages

Judge Points Out Jury Misconduct

By GEORGE NEWMAN
Staff Writer

Citing juror misconduct, a Superior Court judge today

strong feelings about corporations and drug companies "bleeding the public." Allen's decision also

Profits To Black Poor

Muhammad Ali

San Jose News, February 10, 1975

Judge Points Out Jury Misconduct

By GEORGE NEWMAN
Staff Writer

Citing juror misconduct, a Superior Court judge today set aside a $1.1 million award to a 35-year-old San Jose housewife who says she went blind after taking Ortho-Novum birth control pills. The judge also ordered a new trial.

Presiding Judge Bruce F. Allen issued the order after attorneys for the defendants alleged that certain jurors exhibited bias during stages of the trial, which ended in a plaintiff's verdict last Dec. 16.

JURORS' TALK

When informed of the ruling, attorney Sal Liccardo of San Jose, representing Mrs. Michelle Ahearn and her husband, Dennis, said:

"The decision comes as a total shock and surprise."

Liccardo said he immediately intends to appeal Allen's decision.

In his written order, Allen cited irregularity in the proceedings of the jury by which the defendants were prevented from having a fair trial," and "misconduct of the jury."

Specifically, Allen referred to sworn affidavits handed him by defense attorneys in which jurors interviewed by investigators for the defense declared that they were persuaded in arguments by two other jurors which were outside the limits of the judge's instructions.

ATTORNEY'S SHOCK

One of the jurors, Vernon Van Leuven, according to Allen's decision, said the two other jurors, Mrs. Glennys Spitze and Mrs. Marilyn Swanson, told other jurors "they were well informed in relation to medical matters," and "that juror Swanson told the other jurors she had

strong feelings about corporations and drug companies bleeding the public."

Allen's decision also further cited Van Leuven's affidavit in which he alleged that Mrs. Swanson "read to the jurors a prepared statement about big corporations, how much money the drug companies were making, and they should be held responsible."

The decision also cited an affidavit of alternate juror William Stillwell in which Stillwell quoted Mrs. Spitze, who served as the jury's foreman, as discussing lie

(Back of Section, Col. 4)

$1.1 Million Jury Award Wiped Out

(Continued from Page 1)

detector equipment and its relationship to a witness.

She alledgedly told her fellow jurors, according to the affidavit, that because of her familiarity with such testimony and her observations of the witness, that his testimony could not be true.

Stillwell's affidavit also cited a juror lunch in which Mrs. Spitze allegedly compared trial testimony with the experience of her own son's hospitalization.

The irregularity cited by Allen involved a juror, Anthony Astalfa, who voted in favor of the verdicts for both Ahearns, but declined to say, when formally polled whether he agreed that the birth pill was a substantial factor in causing Mrs. Ahearn's blindness.

Allen concluded, "It is probable that a different result would have been reached but for such bias, prejudice and misconduct on the part of these three jurors."

Meanwhile, attorney Liccardo said he had filed affidavits "from all the other jurors denying that they ever heard any of these conversations."

"You have the word of 13 people (including alternates) to that of alternate Stillwell," Liccardo said.

Liccardo further alleged that the testimony in the affidavit of Van Leuven was rebutted by 11 other jurors.

Mrs. Ahearn, who lives with her engineer husband and three children at 3370 Cardin Ave., burst into tears of joy at the verdict awarding her $1,142,506 and $105,668 in damages to her husband.

San Jose Mercury

More Than a Century of Service—1851-1975

FOURTH YEAR, No. 301   SAN JOSE, CALIF., TUESDAY MORNING FEBRUARY 11, 1975 ★★★★

JUDGE REVERSES VERDICT

Blind Woman Loses $1.1 Million Pill Case

By GEORGE NEWMAN
Staff Writer

A blind San Jose housewife's $1.1 million birth control pill damage verdict was overturned by a judge Monday on grounds that jurors in the case were biased and had engaged in misconduct.

Agreeing to a defense motion for a new trial, Presiding Superior Court Judge Bruce F. Allen at the same time signed an order setting aside the jury's award. No new trial date was set.

The amount was fixed last

Related story on Page 17

Dec. 16 by jurors determining damages for Mrs. Michelle Ahearn, a mother of three, and her husband, Dennis, a structural engineer.

Mrs. Ahearn, 35, of 3370 Cardin Ave., sought the damages after sustaining total loss of her sight. She alleged that her blindness was caused, either fully or in part, by a birth control pill, Ortho-Novum, manufactured by Johnson and Johnson.

Following announcement of Allen's decision, the Ahearns' attorney, Sal Liccardo, immediately filed a notice of appeal with the court clerk's office.

"Mrs. Ahearn was shocked and upset by the news," Liccardo said after informing his client of the ruling.

In his written decision, entered in the court record, Allen wrote that he was setting aside the verdicts because of "irregularity in the proceedingss of the jury by which defendants were prevented from having a fair trial," and "misconduct of the jury."

Allen, who presided over the trial, referred specifically to sworn affidavits handed him by defense.

The jurors were interviewed after the trial and after they had been discharged.

Allen wrote that an affidavit by of one of the jurors, Vernon Van Leuven, alleged that two other jurors, Mrs. Glennys Spitze and Mrs. Marilyn Swanson, had told other jurors that "they were well informed in relation to medical matters."

He cited further that Van

(Back of Section, Col. 6)

BIRTH CONTROL CASE

Blind Woman's Win Reversed

(Continued from Page 1)

Leuven's affidavit alleged that Mrs. Swanson "told the other jurors she had strong feelings about corporations and drug companies bleeding the public."

The Van Leuven affidavit also alleged, according to Allen's written decision, that Mrs. Swanson "read to the other jurors a prepared statement about big corporations, how much money the drug companies were making and they should be held responsible."

Allen wrote that an affidavit of alternate juror William Stillwell quoted Mrs. Spitze, who served as jury foreman, as telling fellow jurors that through her familiarity with lie detector processes she was somehow able to determine that the testimony of a defense witness "could not be true."

"Again, this was serious misconduct," Allen wrote.

"I can only conclude that Mrs. Spitze should not have been on the jury because she was an advocate for plaintiff, that she was not impartial, that she was biased for plaintiff from prior experience," Allen wrote.

Allen also cited the alleged irregularity, which involved a juror, Anthony Astalfa, who voted in favor of the unanimous verdicts for both Ahearns. However, Astalfa declined to say, when formally polled at the end of the trial, whether he agreed that the pill was a substantial factor in causing Mrs. Ahearn's blindness.

(A minimum of nine juror votes are needed here for a verdict in a civil trial.)

The verdict had come without apparent dissension among jurors over the matter of causation and amount of damages. Only one juror when polled acknowledged that he could not state that the drug caused Mrs. Ahearn's blindness, a fact dwelt on by Judge Allen in his reversal.

"It is probable that a different result would have been reached but for such bias, prejudice and misconduct on the part of these three jurors," Allen wrote.

Allen's instructions had required that jurors not discuss the case until all testimony was completed and at that point to consider only evidence presented during the trial.

Allen wrote in several pages Monday that he also believed the weight of the evidence clearly favored the defense.

As an example, he cited the expert witness to testimony of a Dr. Overton, a Texas neurosurgeon, who appeared in behalf of Mrs. Ahearn:

"His (Dr. Overton's) demeanor on the witness stand was extremely belligerent, hostile toward defendants, and agitated. He has received high fees for testifying and consulting for various plaintiffs in pill cases."

Allen concluded that "the jury clearly should have reached a different special verdict and different general verdicts — that the special verdict should have been a finding of no causation, that the Ortho-Novum was not a substantial factor in causing plaintiff's blindness," and that "Mrs. Ahearn and her husband receive "nothing on the general verdicts."

Liccardo said that before Allen's decision he had filed affidavits "from all the other jurors denying that they ever heard of any of these conversations."

"You have the word of 13 people (including alternates) to that of Stillwell," Liccardo said.

Liccardo said that the affidavit testimony of Van Leuven was also rebutted by the affidavits of 11 other jurors.

Mrs. Ahearn became suddenly blind in February, 1969, at the same time that she was taking the pill and suffering from a streptococcus infection.

The Ahearns' appeal of Allen's decision will be considered by the District Court of Appeal in San Francisco.

San Jose Mercury News, February 11, 1975—Continued

Tried Their Best, Say Overruled Jurors

"I tried to the best of my ability. I still feel it was a fair decision," said a member of the Santa Clara County Superior Court jury whose $11-million damage award to a blinded San Jose housewife was overturned.

Mrs. Janet M. Hurst of Mountain View was one of only five of the 12-member panel who would talk for publication following announcement of the reversal Monday, but her comments reflected a feeling expressed by others.

Related story on page 1

All of the jurors and the two alternates have their sworn affidavits on file in connection with the motion initiated by attorneys for the three defendant firms involved in the manufacture and sale of a birth control pill that assertedly cost the sight of Mrs. Michelle Ahearn.

These who declined to comment referred the questioner to the court statements.

But Mrs. Hurst and the others were firm in declaring there was no bias or prejudice in their findings as implied in the order signed by Judge Bruce F. Allen based on "irregularity in the proceedings of the jury ... misconduct of the jury, insufficiency of the evidence and excessive damages."

"I think the layman is presented with a huge decision," said Mrs. Hurst. "Perhaps lay people are asked too much."

But until the law is changed, she said, she feels citizens have a duty to serve on juries and she'd serve again herself

Mrs. Carol Morris of Los Gatos said there was "mutual respect -- no pressuring" on the part of jurors in fact, when they returned to begin deliberations on a Thursday afternoon, the jurors "held hands and had prayer," she said.

Jurors, she said, felt a "heavy responsibility.

"It's wrong to say we were biased or prejudiced," Mrs. Morris declared.

Mrs. Joann R. Kauffman of Sunnyvale said she never heard any of the purportedly prejudicial statements. She said the jurors originally were far apart on the question of damages but arrived at a figure on which they all agreed "by compromise."

She noted that the jury had three tasks: to stille the matter of causation, if causation were found, to determine whether it was the result of negligence or breach of contract, and, if there was liability on either of those bases, to fix the amount of damages.

It was the question of causation that brought the opinion of juror Anthony Astalfa into question. Astalfa had concurred with the rest on the amount of damages, but when polled after the verdict, he couldn't say whether the drug was a substantial factor in causing blindness.

He still couldn't say for sure Monday night.

"It could have been proved to me either way," he said, acknowledging that he had agreed with the others on damages.

He said he felt that at the time of the occurrence more than six years ago, manufacturers did not furnish sufficient warning with the pills.

Astalfa denied that he had eaten lunch with other jurors when one of the women panel members had made allegedly prejudicial comments, as had been noted in an affidavit quoted by Judge Allen.

One of the other jurors had suggested that, on the matter of causation, the instruction hadn't been entirely clear, that is, it wasn't made plain that if one wasn't sure about causation, one couldn't rule on the matter of damages.

Judge Allen's ruling indicated otherwise.

Mrs. Philomene Leal of Campbell said she "felt kind of bad" at the reversal.

She too, was firm in her denial of bias or prejudice. "I made up my own mind," Mrs. Leal declared.

Among the jurors commenting there was agreement that the matter of liability was agreed on by the necessary majority of three-fourths (nine jurors) at the outset.

One recalled that "the first time around the table" it was nine to three for liability, then quickly 10 to two. Another recalled the 10 to two as being the initial polling.

'Retrial By Affidavit' Drawing Fire

By GEORGE NEWMAN
Staff Writer

The question whether limits should exist for investigators probing post-trial juror details arose here Tuesday in the wake of a judge's order reversing the verdict in a major birth control pill case.

While the judge in the case declined to comment beyond his written ruling, others in the valley's legal community expressed their views, including a former bar official who urged abolishing the privilege.

Those who commented were reacting to a ruling Monday in which Presiding Superior Court Judge Bruce F. Allen overturned a blind San Jose housewife's $1.1-million damage verdict on grounds that jurors in the case were biased and had engaged in misconduct.

And the private investigator who interviewed most of the trial jurors following the verdict, himself declined to comment, citing the need to maintain "fairness" to his client.

Recipients of the jury award, set aside Monday by Allen, were Mrs. Michelle Ahearn, 35, and her husband, Dennis, a structural engineer.

Allen, also ordered a new trial in the case. His decision is being appealed.

The investigator, Scott Newby, of 4036 Valerie Drive, Campbell, confirmed that he had been hired by Johnson and Johnson, manufacturers of the birth control pill, Ortho-Novum, to interview jurors in the case.

"In fairness to my client, I can't comment beyond that at this time," Newby said. "Perhaps at a later date."

Newby had contacted The Mercury several weeks ago, seeking additional information about juror courtroom actions following reading of the verdict.

He was routinely referred to the newspaper's published account of the trial.

Attorney Conrad Rushing, imediate past president of the Santa Clara County Bar Association, said he believed that Allen applied the law in the case, but he took issue with the system that allows what he termed "a re-trial of a case by affidavit."

Rushing referred to juror affidavits furnished to judges by lawyers that purport to show misconduct, or willful disregard of instructions by other jurors.

"I think that part of the system is wrong and it's bad policy," Rushing declared. "I think we ought to get rid of that part of the system."

Rushing said that in early America jurors were expected to take with them into the jury room their prior experiences and prejudices.

"The law as it is being applied today requires that jurors' minds must be seen as the cleanest blackboard, and that probably is an impossible thing to find," Rushing said.

"For example, one of the affidavits (in the birth control pill case) said that one of the jurors felt that the drug companies in the United States were overreaching in terms of price and marketing, and that seems to be a view that is held by a number of national leaders and seems to be a view widely held in the community," said Rushing.

"To say that in itself makes the juror incapable of judging events is to prevent the person from serving because they hold a political or economic belief," Rushing said.

Two Superior Court judges were asked whether the decision might signal the start of a lawyer trend to reopen cases by bringing forth details of jury room deliberations, heretofore believed by most of the public to be secret.

The judges, John S. McInerny and Peter Anello, both emphasized that jurors are under no obligation to discuss their jury room deliberation after they have been discharged from duty.

"I tell my jurors that they need not discuss the case with anyone unless they wish to do so," Anello said.

While both Anello and McInery said that thought that they had not been faced with a similar situation in their combined 22 years on the bench, they agreed that Allen holds the legal discretion to exercise much an order.

According to McInerny, it was in years past a practiced use that a jury verdict could not be impeached. However, a 1959 U.S. Supreme Court decision allows certain juror issues, such as the misconduct allegations raised in the birth control pill case, to be resented to the trial judge.

What will be the reaction of the citizenry if they realize that anything said in the secrecy of the jury room deliberations might at a later time be made fully public, McInerny was asked.

"I really believe that jury deliberations must remain secret, but at the same time, if something blatantly went on, the attorneys should be able to bring it to the attention of the trial judge," McInery replied.

A prominent defense attorney, who asked that his name not be printed, said it is virtually standard practice among defense lawyers to pay a $300 investigation fee for brief interviews of jurors, following a jury trial in which a plaintiff's verdict is returned. The same often holds true for plaintiff's lawyers, he added.

Only in instances where apparent juror misconduct or bias surfaces does there follow a more intensive and detailed investigation, he said.

The Mercury
★★★★   SAN JOSE, CALIF., WEDNESDAY, FEBRUARY 12, 1975   72

SAN JOSE NEWS

S.J. pill edict reversed

$1 MILLION AWARD

Blinded woman wins

By GEORGE NEWMAN
Staff Writer

Blind San Jose housewife Michelle Ahearn, whose $1.1 million birth control pill damage verdict was overturned by a judge, won her case on appeal today.

The damage award, made more than two years ago, now stands, and the judge's order setting asidethe jury verdict is overturned.

In a unanimous ruling, the District Court of Appeal reversed a decision by Santa Clara County Superior Judge Bruce F. Allen, who had earlier declared the award improper on several grounds.

One of the grounds was alleged juror misconduct, stemming from an accusation by defense attorneys that jurors made prejudicial remarks during their deliberations.

The three-judge appeals panel, in affirming the earlier jury verdict, declared that even assuming the truth of certain juror reports about what was discussed it could "observe no substantial misconduct."

"The claimed remarks were made during the jury's deliberations, and were consistent with . . . strong feelings about corporations and drug companies." the decision read in part.

Mrs. Ahearn, 37, mother of three children, was awarded the large sum on Dec. 16, 1974, after a six-week trial.

Mrs. Ahearn, of 3370 Cardin Ave., began taking Ortho-novum, manufactured by Ortho Pharmceutical Co., a subsidiary of Johnson & Johnson, back in 1967 on her doctor's perscription.

She testified she suffered periodic headaches while taking the pills and in 1969 started to experience the onset of blindness.

Doctors said her blindness was

San Jose News, March 18, 1977

San Jose woman's appeal worth $1 million damages

(Continued from Page 1)

caused by clots which blocked the supply of blood to her optic nerves, causing them to atrophy.

Attorney Sal Liccardo, who represented Mrs. Ahearn, said his client received the news with great enthusiasm.

He quoted her as saying she "had faith that the jury's decision would be upheld."

At the time, Allen also ruled that, in his opinion, the weight of the evidence clearly favored the defense. In its decision today the appellate panel found "no substantial basis in the record for the trial court's (Allen's) stated rea-

sons for granting a new trial on the ground of insufficiency of the evidence."

The panel members are Presiding Justice John B. Molinari, and Associate Justices Richard Sims Sr. and Norman Elkington.

Commenting on Allen's acceptance of declarations from jurors and alternate jurors, the panel declared taking of such "hearsay statements" improper.

As a consequence of the decision, Allen's order setting aside the jury verdict and granting a new trial was overturned and the award stands. Only an appeal to the California Supreme Court remains for the drug firm.

Meanwhile, in the downtown courtroom of Superior Court Judge Albert DeMarco, a jury today refused to award damages to a woman who took the same birth control pill, claiming it resulted severe brain damage.

The woman, Mrs. Dorothy Louise Curran, 38, of Seattle, Wash., used the pill in 1974 after which she suffered the impairment.

Her lawyer contended she suffered a stroke due to blood clots resulting from the pill, while the defense alleged she was the victim of a disease. Her lawyer in the case also was Liccardo.

San Jose News, **March 18, 1977—Continued**

The Mercury News

SAN JOSE, CALIFORNIA, SATURDAY MORNING, MARCH 19, 1977

17A

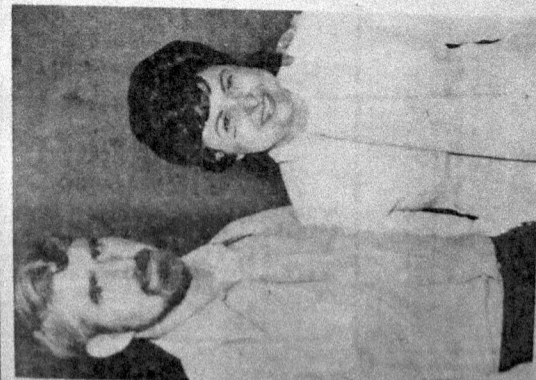

Michelle Ahearn, husband Dennis, show joy at appeal court decision

EARLIER VERDICT REVERSED

$1.1 Million For Blinded Woman

By GEORGE NEWMAN
Staff Writer

An appellate court Friday ordered payment of a $1.1 million jury damage award to a San Jose housewife who lost her eyesight after taking birth control pills.

The ruling in the case of Mrs. Michelle Ahearn overturned an earlier decision by Santa Clara County Superior Court Judge Bruce F. Allen, who had set aside the large award.

For Mrs. Ahearn, 37, mother of three children, the higher court ruling may have ended an ordeal that began in 1967, when she began taking Ortho-Novum, a birth pill manufactured by a subsidiary of Johnson & Johnson.

She suffered periodic headaches while taking the pills until 1969, when she experienced the onset of blindness, caused by clots, which blocked the supply of blood to her optic nerves.

On Dec. 16, 1974, a Superior Court jury unanimously awarded $1.1 million to Mrs. Ahearn, who lives with her family at 3370 Cardin Ave.

However, a few weeks later, Judge Allen ordered the jury's award set aside on grounds of juror misconduct and that the verdict was not justified by the evidence.

Allen had accepted affidavits presented by defense lawyers alleging that some jurors had told other jurors that they were well informed about medical matters. Another juror was quoted as saying she had

strong feelings about corporations and drug companies "bleeding the public."

In this decision reversing Allen, the three-judge panel declared it could find no basis for Allen's granting a new trial on the ground of insufficient evidence.

It also declared "improper" Allen's allowing of hearsay statements of jurors in avidavits presented to him by defense lawyers following the trial.

However, the panel noted, even assuming the truth of the juror allegations, "we observe no substantial misconduct."

The appellate panel members were Presiding Justice John Molinari and Justices Richard Sims and Norman Elkington.

Mrs. Ahearn wasn't immediately available for comment, but her lawyer, Sal Liccardo, said she told him when she learned the news that the ruling "reaffirms her faith in the system of justice."

Liccardo said the last two years, while awaiting outcome of the appeal, "had been very depressing" to Mrs. Ahearn and her husband, Dennis, a structural engineer.

The appellate decision also met with comment from Mrs. Glenny Spitze of Morgan Hill, who served as foreman of the jury which returned the $1.1 million verdict.

In a written decision tossing out the jury verdict (following the trial), Allen ruled that Mrs. Spitze "should not have been on the jury because she was an advocate for plaintiff, that she was not impartial, that she was biased for plaintiff from prior experience."

When contacted by a reporter, Mrs. Spitze said she felt that both the jury system as well as her own personal actions had been vindicated by the appellate decision.

She added: "I couldn't believe that when there were 12 jurors who unanimously decided on something . . . a judge could do something like this. We had tried very hard to do the right thing and follow all the rules. I felt we were used by the judge and the drug companies."

Earlier this year, the California Supreme Court had ruled similarly on a Southern California case, in which it commented that if in the future lawyers were to be permitted to bring to a court's attention discussions occurring during juror deliberations, there would result an unwillingness on the part of citizens to serve.

As a consequence of Friday's ruling Allen's earlier order setting aside the jury verdict and granting a new trial has been overturned. The original jury award stands, and only a possible appeal to the State Supreme Court could alter the status.

Meanwhile, another Santa Clara County Superior Court jury Friday refused to award damages to a woman who took Ortho-Novum, claiming it resulted in severe brain damage.

Medical witnesses testified that Mrs. Dorothy Curran, 38, of Seattle, Wash., suffered a stroke after using the pill in 1974, but defense experts contended that her impairment resulted from a brain disease. Her lawyer in the case was also Liccardo.

10   San Jose Mercury Tuesday, June 14, 1977

Woman Blinded By The Pill To Keep $1.1-Million Award

By GEORGE NEWMAN
Staff Writer

Michelle Ahearn, the San Jose housewife who lost her eyesight after taking birth-control pills, has won the deciding round in an appeal battle over her $1.1-million damage award.

The California Supreme Court, in denying a petition for hearing, upheld the damage award returned by a Superior Court jury here.

A Supreme Court spokesman in San Francisco said two justices, William Clark and Frank Richardson, voted to hear the case, while Chief Justice Rose Bird and Justices Mathew Tobriner, Wiley Manuel and Stanley Mosk dissented.

Four affirmative votes are required to grant a petition for hearing.

The hearing was sought by the defendant in the case, Johnson & Johnson, manufacturer of the birth control pill Ortho-Novum, in an attempt to overturn a ruling by the state's First District Court of Appeal.

The three-judge appellate court

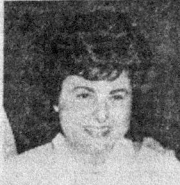

MICHELLE AHEARN
. . . Glad it's over

unanimously decided last March 18 that Santa Clara County Superior Court Judge Bruce F. Allen wrongfully took away the award from Mrs. Ahearn, mother of three children.

The appellate panel reversed Judge Allen's decision setting aside the jury's verdict and granting a new trial in the matter.

Judge Allen delivered his ruling a few weeks after a jury on Dec.

16, 1974 unanimously awarded $1.1 million to Mrs. Ahearn.

According to Mrs. Ahearn's attorney, Sal Liccardo, the high court decision ends the case.

"There is no legal ground for taking the case to the U.S. Supreme Court. The matter is final," Liccardo said.

The decision marked the last chapter in an ordeal that began for the 37-year-old mother when she began taking Ortho-Novum in 1967.

She suffered periodic headaches while taking the pills until 1969, when she experienced the onset of blindness, caused by clots, which blocked the supply of blood of her optic nerves.

Though Mrs. Ahearn or her husband Dennis, a structural engineer, were not immediately available for comment, the couple issued the following statement through their lawyer.

"We are relieved to learn of the decision. We can't believe that finally, after eight years, it is over."

Liccardo said the couple hoped they could soon return to a normal life.

Although the jury that awarded Mrs. Ahearn the $1.1 million was unanimous in its verdict, Judge Allen ordered the jury's verdict set aside on grounds of juror misconduct and that the evidence did not justify the verdict.

Judge Allen had accepted affidavits presented by defense lawyers alleging that some jurors had told other jurors that they were well-informed about medical matters. Another juror was quoted in the affidavits as saying she had strong feelings about corporations and companies "bleeding the public."

In its subsequent decision reversing Judge Allen, the District Court of Appeal declared in a written ruling that it could find no basis for granting a new trial. It also found no substantial evidence of juror misconduct, and ordered that the jury verdict be allowed to stand.

After the District Court of Appeal's reversal of Judge Allen's decision, the drug firm took the case to the state Supreme Court seeking to overturn the appellate court's decision.

Appendix A

<u>GLOSSARY</u>

VEIN -   a blood vessel that returns used blood from body tissues toward the heart.

ARTERY -   a blood vessel that takes blood from the heart to the body tissues.

THROMBUS -   a blood clot formed within either a vein or an artery, or in a chamber of the heart.

THROMBOSIS -   the process of formation of a thrombus (or <u>thrombi</u> [plural]).

THROMBOPHLEBITIS -   blood clots within veins associated with inflammation of the vein walls.

THROMBOEMBOLIC -   refers to clots within blood vessels and/or movement of those clots (embolism) to parts of the body away from the part where they formed.

INFLAMMATION -   reaction of body tissues to injury.

CELLULITIS -   inflammation of loose tissues, such as that just beneath the skin.

ORBITAL CELLULITIS - inflammation of the loose tissues of the orbit (the bony cavity containing the eyeball).

CAVERNOUS SINUS -   a blood channel (in the system of veins) situated deep in the skull, just behind the two orbits; blood flows into it from veins in the orbits.

CAVERNOUS SINUS
THROMBOSIS -   blood clot within the cavernous sinus.

OPHTHALMIC VEINS -   veins that drain blood from the eye, back into the Cavernous Sinus.

PATHOLOGY -   branch of medical science that deals with the nature of disease, particularly changes in tissues caused by disease.

OPHTHALMOLOGY -   branch of medical science that deals with diagnosis and treatment of disorders of the eye.

OTOLARYNGOLOGY -   branch of medical science that deals with diagnosis and treatment of disorders of the ears, nose and throat.

APPENDIX "A-1"

Medical Glossary Given to Jurors

NEUROLOGY -	branch of medical science that deals with the diagnosis and treatment of physical disorders of the nervous system.
NEUROSURGERY -	branch of medical science that deals with the diagnosis and surgical treatment of certain disorders of the nervous system.
EPIDEMIOLOGY -	science of the study of causes, distribution, and frequencies of diseases in humans.
PHARMACOLOGY -	branch of medical science that deals with the effects of drugs on humans and animals.
HEMATOLOGY -	branch of medical science that deals with diagnosis and treatment of diseases of the blood and blood-forming organs.
RADIOLOGY -	branch of medical science that deals with the use of X-rays in medical diagnosis and treatment.
ORTHO-NOVUM -	brand of birth control pills consumed by Plaintiff Michelle Ahearn. It consists of two synthetic hormones.
PROGESTIN or PROGESTOGEN -	a synthetic hormone which acts like the natural female hormone progesterone, one of those produced by the ovary.
ESTROGEN -	a general term for another classification of female hormones produced naturally by a woman's ovary, or made synthetically.
NORETHINDRONE -	the progestin component of Ortho-Novum.
MESTRANOL -	the estrogen component of Ortho-Novum.
P.D.R. -	abbreviation for Physicians' Desk Reference, a book published and distributed without charge every year to all practicing physicians in the United States; it contains information on prescription drugs.

APPENDIX "A-2"

Medical Glossary Given to Jurors—Continued

F.D.A. -   abbreviation for the Food and Drug Administration.

C.V.A. -   abbreviation for Cerebro-Vascular Accident,
                          a synonym for "stroke."

EDEMA -   abnormal swelling of tissues of the body.

ANGIOGRAM -   an X-ray study of blood vessels, made by
                          injecting a "dye" into the bloodstream before
                          taking X-ray pictures.

ARTERIOGRAM -   an angiogram of arteries.

VENOGRAM -   an angiogram of veins.

MENINGITIS -   inflammation of the meninges, the membranes
                          which cover and brain and line the skull.

STREPTOCOCCUS -   one of the common types of germs (bacteria)
                          which may cause infection.

PACKAGE INSERT -   a printed document containing the "official"
                          information about the use of a prescription
                          drug, and accompanying packages of the drug
                          going to pharmacists and to physicians.

BLOOD CULTURE -   a laboratory procedure for discovering bacteria
                          in the bloodstream.

APPENDIX "A-3"

Medical Glossary Given to Jurors—Continued

ACKNOWLEDGMENTS

I first owe a debt of gratitude to Michelle and Dennis Ahearn for not only allowing me to write and publish this work that is so personal to their lives, but even more so for their courage in allowing me to pursue the case from the beginning to the end—a true search for the truth for them.

For their advice, assistance, and continued encouragement to write and complete this work, a very special thanks to my wife, Laura; my children, Rosalie and her husband Joe; Laura; Sam and his wife Jessica; Paul and his wife Toni, and my grandson, Jason and his wife Jessica. To the many trial lawyers and close friends who constantly commented when they heard this story,

"You need to write a book," I am grateful.

I am particularly indebted to my paralegal and trial assistant for over 30 years, Katy Buompensiero, for her hard work and dedication in editing both language and substance from the beginning of the book to the end, and also to Nicole Buompensiero for her linguistic talents in assisting Katy in preparing the work for publication.

Last but not least, without the incredible contributions of all of those identified within this book who were an essential part of the story, most especially Dr. Harold Williams, there never would have been a story to be told.